ENT

AN INTRODUCTION
AND PRACTICAL GUIDE

EDITED BY

James Russell Tysome MA PhD FRCS (ORL-HNS)
Senior Clinical Fellow in Neurotology and Skull Base Surgery
Cambridge University Hospitals NHS Foundation Trust

AND

Rahul Govind Kanegaonkar FRCS (ORL-HNS)
Consultant ENT Surgeon
Medway NHS Foundation Trust
Guy's and St Thomas' NHS Foundation Trust

HODDER ARNOLD

First published in Great Britain in 2012 by
Hodder Arnold, an imprint of Hodder Education, Hodder and Stoughton Ltd,
a division of Hachette UK
338 Euston Road, London NW1 3BH

http://www.hodderarnold.com

Hachette UK's policy is to use papers that are natural, renewable and recyclable
products and made from wood grown in sustainable forests. The logging and
manufacturing processes are expected to conform to the environmental regulations
of the country of origin.

Whilst the advice and information in this book are believed to be true and accurate at
the date of going to press, neither the author[s] nor the publisher can accept any legal
responsibility or liability for any errors or omissions that may be made. In particular,
(but without limiting the generality of the preceding disclaimer) every effort has been
made to check drug dosages; however it is still possible that errors have been missed.
Furthermore, dosage schedules are constantly being revised and new side-effects
recognized. For these reasons the reader is strongly urged to consult the drug
companies' printed instructions, and their websites, before administering any of
the drugs recommended in this book.

British Library Cataloguing in Publication Data
A catalogue record for this book is available from the British Library

Library of Congress Cataloging-in-Publication Data
A catalog record for this book is available from the Library of Congress

ISBN-13   978-1-444-14908-1

1 2 3 4 5 6 7 8 9 10

Commissioning Editor: Francesca Naish
Production Controller: Joanna Walker
Cover Design: Helen Townson
Project management provided by Naughton Project Management

Typeset in 10/12 pt Minion Regular by Datapage
Printed and bound in Spain by Graphycems

What do you think about this book? Or any other Hodder Arnold title?
Please visit our website: www.hodderarnold.com

Dedication
This book is dedicated to Dipalee, Amee and Deven
and to Laura, George and Henry

CONTENTS

CONTRIBUTORS

Mr Ketan Desai FRCS
Associate Specialist in Otorhinolaryngology
Royal Sussex County Hospital, Brighton

Mr Neil Donnelly MSc (Hons) FRCS (ORL-HNS)
Consultant Otoneurological and Skull Base Surgeon
Cambridge University Hospitals NHS Foundation Trust

Dr Dipalee Vijay Durve MRCPCH FRCR
Consultant Radiologist
Guy's and St Thomas' NHS Foundation Trust

Mr Steven Frampton MA MRCS DOHNS
ENT Specialist Trainee Registrar
Wessex Region

Mr Jonathan Hughes MRCS DOHNS
Specialist Registrar in Otolaryngology
North Thames rotation/Royal National Throat Nose and Ear Hospital

Mr Ram Moorthy FRCS (ORL-HNS)
Consultant ENT Surgeon
Heatherwood and Wexham Park Hospitals NHS Foundation Trust
and Honorary Consultant ENT Surgeon, Northwick Park Hospital

Ms Joanne Rimmer FRCS (ORL-HNS)
Specialist Registrar in Otolaryngology
North Thames rotation/Royal National Throat Nose and Ear Hospital

Mr Francis Vaz FRCS (ORL-HNS)
Consultant ENT/Head and Neck Surgeon
University College London Hospital

FOREWORD

The 'Introduction to ENT' course has now become an established and must attend course for the novice ENT practitioner. The synergistic blend of didactic teaching and practical skills training has allowed many junior trainees to raise the standard of care they deliver to their ENT patients.

The course manual is now a 'Bible' for juniors in nursing and medicine caring for patients on the wards, clinics or in emergency room. The Royal College of Surgeons has endorsed this course in the past and it continues to maintain a high standard of post graduate training. I would strongly recommend this course to any trainee embarking on a career in ENT.

Khalid Ghufoor

Otolaryngology Tutor
Raven Department of Education
The Royal College of Surgeons of England

PREFACE

This book has been written for trainees in otorhinolaryngology and to update general practitioners. Common and significant pathology that might present itself is described. Included also are relevant supporting specialties such as audiology and radiology. A significant proportion of this text has been devoted to common surgical procedures, their indications and operative techniques, as well as the management of their complications. We do hope that the text will facilitate and encourage junior trainees to embark on a career in this diverse and rewarding specialty.

Writing this book would not have been possible had it not been for the encouragement of our many friends and colleagues, and the unfaltering support of our families.

We would, however, like to make a special mention of some extraordinary and gifted tutors without whom we may not have initiated the popular 'Introduction to ENT' course nor written the course manual from which this text originates. Ghassan Alusi, Alec Fitzgerald O'Connor, Khalid Ghufoor, Govind Kanegaonkar, Robert Tranter and the late Roger Parker instilled in us a passion for teaching, nurtured our curiosity for all things medical and encouraged us to undertake the research that has served us so well.

INTRODUCTION

Otorhinolaryngology (ENT) is a diverse and challenging specialty which is poorly represented on the busy Medical School curriculum. Although an estimated 20% of cases seen in primary care are ENT-related, many general practitioners have little or no direct clinical training in this field.

This book has evolved from the *Introduction to ENT* course manual which has served so many of us so well. Over 1200 doctors have attended this course and its *Essential Guide* partner over the last eight years.

This book covers both common and the life-threatening emergencies that may present in primary care. It not only describes the common management pathways for conditions, but also lists possible complications of procedures and their treatment and provides a basis for referral if there is doubt.

The updated colour illustrations concisely depict relevant clinical anatomy without unduly simplifying the topic in question.

I am certain this text will prove to be as, if not more, popular and relevant to general practitioners than the *Introduction to ENT* text from which it is derived.

Dr Junaid Bajwa
June 2011

CLINICAL ANATOMY

THE EAR

The ear is divided into three separate but related subunits. The outer ear consists of the pinna and external auditory canal bounded medially by the lateral surface of the tympanic membrane. The middle ear contains the ossicular chain, which spans the middle ear cleft and allows acoustic energy to be transferred from the tympanic membrane to the oval window and hence the cochlea of the inner ear.

This elaborate mechanism has evolved to overcome the loss of acoustic energy that occurs when transferring sound from one medium to another (impedance mismatch), in this case from air to fluid.

▌ The outer ear

The pinna consists largely of elastic cartilage over which the skin is tightly adherent (Figure 1.1). The cartilage is dependent on the overlying perichondrium for its nutritional support; hence separation of this layer from the cartilage by a haematoma, abscess or inflammation secondary to piercing may result in cartilage necrosis resulting in permanent deformity (cauliflower ear). The lobule, in contrast, is a fibro-fatty skin tag.

The pinna develops from six mesodermal condensations, the hillocks of His, during the sixth week of embryological development. Three arise from each

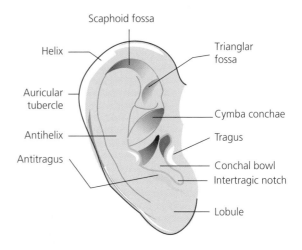

Figure 1.1. Surface landmarks of the pinna.

of the first and second branchial arches on either side of the first pharyngeal groove. These fuse and rotate to produce an elaborate but surprisingly consistent structure. Failure of fusion may result in an accessory auricle or preauricular sinus, while failure of development of the antihelix (from the fourth hillock) in a protruding ('bat') ear.

The external auditory canal is a tortuous passage that directs and redistributes sound from the conchal bowl to the tympanic membrane. The skin of the lateral third of the external auditory canal is thick, contains ceruminous glands, is hair-bearing and tightly adherent to the underlying fibrocartilage. The skin of the medial two-thirds is thin, hairless, tightly bound to underlying bone and exquisitely sensitive.

The sensory nerve supply of the canal is provided by the auriculotemporal and greater auricular nerves. There are minor contributions from the facial nerve (hence vesicles arise on the posterolateral surface of the canal in Ramsay Hunt syndrome) and Arnold's nerve, a branch of the vagus nerve (provoking the cough reflex when stimulated with a cotton bud or during microsuction). The squamous epithelium of the tympanic membrane and ear canal is unique and deserves a special mention. The superficial layer of keratin of the skin of the ear is shed laterally during maturation. This produces an escalator mechanism that allows debris to be directed out of the canal. Disruption of this mechanism may result in debris accumulation, recurrent infections (otitis externa) or erosion of the ear canal, as seen in keratitis obturans.

The tympanic membrane is continuous with the posterior wall of the ear canal and consists of three layers: laterally, a squamous epithelial layer; a middle layer of collagen fibres; and a medial surface lined with respiratory epithelium continuous with the middle ear.

The tympanic membrane is divided into the pars tensa and pars flaccida, or attic (Figure 1.2). They are structurally and functionally different.

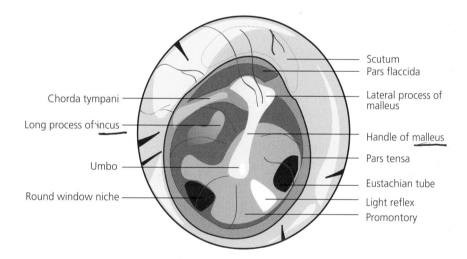

Figure 1.2. Right tympanic membrane.

The collagen fibres of the middle layer of the pars tensa are arranged as lateral radial fibres and medial circumferential fibres that distort the membrane. As a result, the pars tensa 'billows' laterally from the malleus. In contrast, the collagen fibres of the pars flaccida are randomly scattered and this section is relatively flat.

Whilst the surface area of the tympanic membrane of an adult is approximately 80 mm^2, the pars tensa accounts for 55 mm^2. Unlike the pars flaccida, the pars tensa buckles when presented with sound, conducting acoustic energy to the ossicular chain. Interestingly, high-frequency sounds preferentially distort the posterior half of the tympanic membrane, while low-frequency sounds distort the anterior half.

The handle and lateral process of the malleus are embedded within the tympanic membrane and are clearly visible on otoscopy. The long process of the incus is also commonly seen, although the heads of the ossicles are hidden behind the scutum superiorly.

▌ The middle ear

The middle ear is an irregular, air-filled space that communicates with the nasopharynx via the

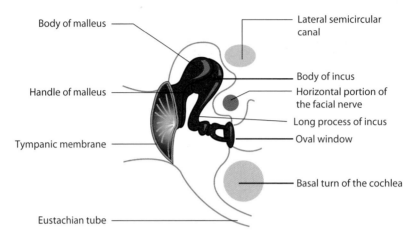

Body of malleus

Handle of malleus

Tympanic membrane

Eustachian tube

Lateral semicircular canal

Body of incus

Horizontal portion of the facial nerve

Long process of incus

Oval window

Basal turn of the cochlea

Figure 1.3. Coronal section of the ossicles in the middle ear.

Eustachian tube (Figure 1.3). Chewing, swallowing and yawning result in untwisting of the tube, allowing air to pass into the middle ear cleft. In children, Eustachian tube dysfunction is common and may result in negative middle ear pressure, recurrent otitis media or middle ear effusions.

The middle ear mechanisms that improve sound transfer include:

- The relative ratios of the areas of the tympanic membrane to stapes footplate (17:1).
- The relative lengths of the handle of malleus to the long process of incus (1.3:1).
- The natural resonance of the outer and middle ears.
- The phase difference between the oval and round windows.
- The buckling effect of the tympanic membrane.

Acoustic energy is conducted by the middle ear ossicles and transferred to the cochlea through the stapes footplate at the oval window. Fixation

of the footplate in otosclerosis prevents sound conduction to the inner ear, resulting in a conductive hearing loss.

▌ The inner ear

The inner ear consists of the cochlea and peripheral vestibular apparatus (Figure 1.4).

The cochlea is a 2¾-turn snail shell that houses the organ of Corti. Acoustic energy causes buckling of the basilar membrane, with deflection maximal at a frequency-specific region of the cochlea. This results in depolarization of the inner hair cells in this region, with information relayed centrally via the cochlear nerve. The cochlea is tonotopic, with high-frequency sounds detected at the basal turn of the cochlea, while low-frequency sounds are detected at the apex.

The peripheral vestibular system is responsible for detecting static, linear and angular head movements. While the semicircular canals are responsible

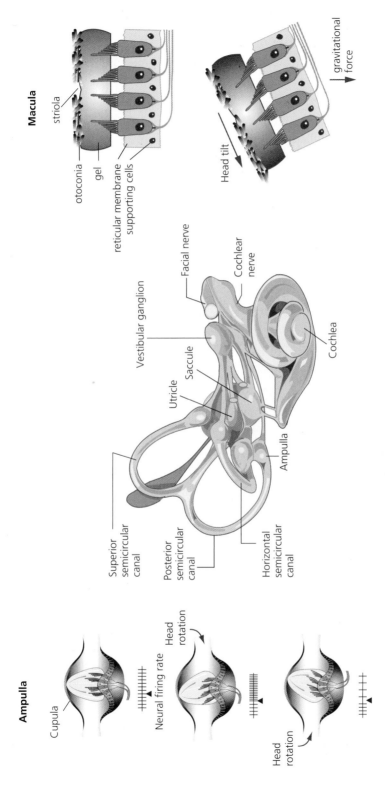

Macula

- striola
- otoconia
- gel
- reticular membrane
- supporting cells

Head tilt

gravitational force

Vestibular ganglion

Facial nerve

Cochlear nerve

Saccule

Utricle

Cochlea

Ampulla

Superior semicircular canal

Posterior semicircular canal

Horizontal semicircular canal

Ampulla

Cupula

Head rotation

Neural firing rate

Head rotation

Figure 1.4. The inner ear. Angular acceleration is detected by the ampullae of the semicircular canals, while linear acceleration and static head tilt are detected by the maculae of the utricle and saccule.

for detecting head rotation, the saccule and utricle are responsible for detecting static head tilt and linear acceleration head tilt. This is achieved by two similar, but functionally different sensory receptor systems (Figure 1.4).

The semicircular canals are oriented in orthogonal planes to one another and organized into functional pairs: the two horizontal semicircular canals; the superior canal and the contralateral posterior canal; and the posterior canal and the contralateral superior canal.

The sensory neuroepithelium of the semicircular canals is limited to a dilated segment of the bony and membranous labyrinth, the ampulla. A crest perpendicular to the long axis of each canal bears a mound of connective tissue from which project a layer of hair cells. Their cilia insert into a gelatinous mass, the cupula, which is deflected during rotational head movements.

The sensory neuroepithelium, responsible for detecting linear acceleration, is limited to specific regions, the maculae. Whilst the macula of the saccule is oriented principally to detect linear acceleration and head tilt in the vertical plane, the macula of the utricle detects linear acceleration and head tilt in the horizontal plane. The hair cells of the maculae are arranged in an elaborate manner and project into a fibro-calcareous sheet, the otoconial membrane. As this membrane has a greater specific gravity than the surrounding endolymph, head tilt and linear movement result in the otoconial membrane moving relative to the underlying hair cells. The shearing force produced causes depolarization of the underlying hair cells with conduction centrally via the vestibular nerve.

THE FACIAL NERVE

The facial nerve (CN VII) has a long and tortuous course through the temporal bone before exiting the skull base at the stylomastoid foramen and passing into the parotid gland (Figure 1.5). Disease processes affecting the inner ear, middle ear, skull base or parotid gland may result in facial nerve paralysis.

The facial nerve arises from the pons and passes laterally as two nerves: facial motor and nervus intermedius. These enter the internal auditory canal where they combine to form the facial nerve. The nerve passes laterally (meatal segment), then anteriorly (labyrinthine section) and within the bony wall of the middle ear undergoes a posterior deflection (the first genu) where the geniculate ganglion is found and the greater petrosal nerve given off (this enters the middle cranial fossa). The facial nerve passes posteriorly (horizontal portion) within the medial wall of the middle ear and then inferiorly (vertical segment) within the temporal bone to exit the skull base at the stylomastoid foramen. During its descent it gives off the chorda tympani nerve, which passes forward and upward entering the middle ear. An additional motor branch supplies the stapedius muscle.

Having left the skull base, the facial nerve gives off branches to the rudimentary muscles of the pinna and a small branch to the external auditory canal. It then continues forward, lying in the tympanomastoid groove to enter the parotid gland, where it divides into superior and inferior divisions before terminating in its five motor branches (Figure 1.6). Additional branches supply the posterior belly of digastric and stylohyoid muscles.

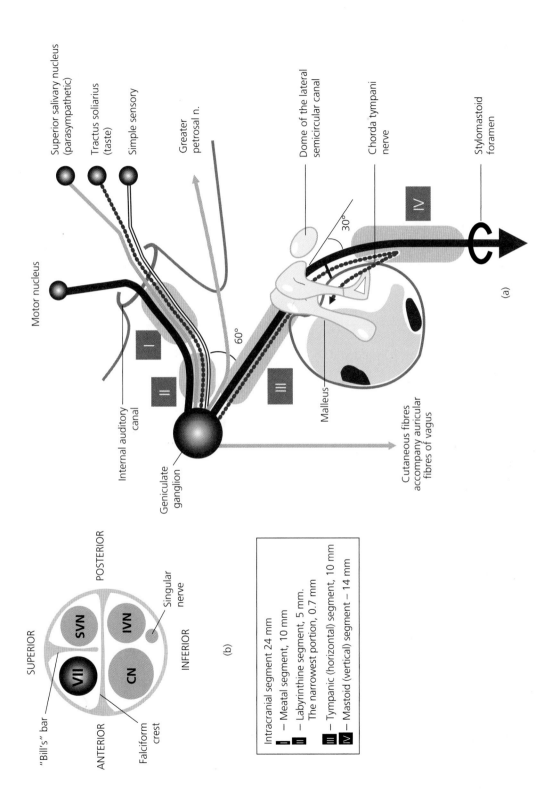

Figure 1.5. The intratemporal course of the facial nerve (a), relative positions of the facial, cochlear and vestibular nerves within the internal auditory canal. (VII = facial nerve, SNV = superior vestibular nerve, IVN = inferior vestibular nerve)

Superior salivary nucleus (parasympathetic)

Tractus soliarius (taste)

Simple sensory

Greater petrosal n.

Dome of the lateral semicircular canal

Chorda tympani nerve

Stylomastoid foramen

Motor nucleus

Internal auditory canal

Geniculate ganglion

Malleus

Cutaneous fibres accompany auricular fibres of vagus

(a)

60°

30°

I

II

III

IV

SUPERIOR

POSTERIOR

"Bill's" bar

SVN

Singular nerve

VII

IVN

ANTERIOR

Falciform crest

CN

INFERIOR

(b)

Intracranial segment 24 mm
– Meatal segment, 10 mm
– Labyrinthine segment, 5 mm.
  The narrowest portion, 0.7 mm
– Tympanic (horizontal) segment, 10 mm
– Mastoid (vertical) segment – 14 mm

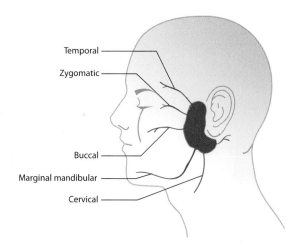

Figure 1.6. External branches of the facial nerve.

THE NOSE

The principal function of the nose is respiration, secondary functions include:

- Warming of inspired air.
- Humidification of inspired air.
- Filtering of large particulate matter by coarse hairs (the vibrisiae) in the nasal vestibule.
- Mucus production, trapping and ciliary clearance of particulate matter.
- Immune protection.
- Olfaction.
- Drainage/aeration of the middle ear cleft via the Eustachian tube.
- Drainage/aeration of the paranasal sinuses.
- Drainage for the nasolacrimal duct.
- Prevention of lung alveolar collapse via the nasal cycle.
- Voice modification.
- Pheromone detection via the Vomero-nasal organ of Jacobsen.

▮ Nasal skeleton

The external nasal skeleton consists of bone in the upper third (the nasal bones) and cartilage in the lower two-thirds. External nasal landmarks are illustrated in Figure 1.7.

The upper aero-digestive tract is divided into the nasal cavity, oral cavity, oropharynx, larynx and hypopharynx (Figure 1.8).

▮ The nasal cavities

The nasal cavities are partitioned in the midline by the nasal septum, which consists of both fibrocartilage and bone (Figure 1.9).

As with the cartilage of the pinna, the cartilage of the septum is dependent on the overlying adherent perichondrium for its nutritional support. Separation of this layer by haematoma or abscess may result in cartilage necrosis and a saddle nose cosmetic deformity.

The venous drainage of the nose and mid-face communicates with the cavernous sinus of the middle cranial fossa via the ophthalmic veins, deep facial vein and pterygoid plexus. As a result, an infection in this territory may spread intracranially, resulting in cavernous sinus thrombosis and death.

In contrast to the smooth surface of the nasal septum, the lateral wall is thrown into folds by three

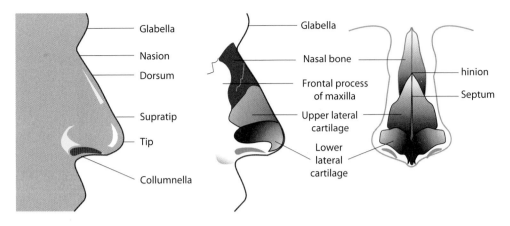

Figure 1.7. Nasal landmarks and external nasal skeleton.

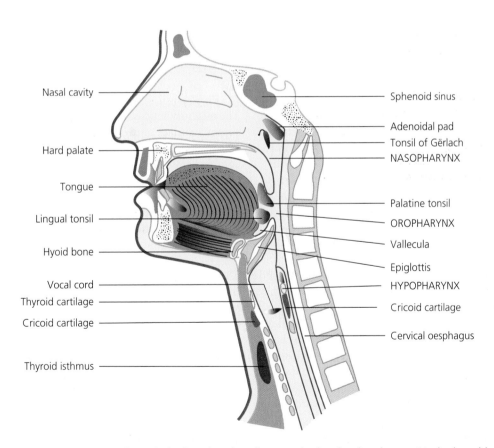

Figure 1.8. Sagittal section through the head and neck. Note the hard palate lies at C1, the hyoid bone at C3 and the cricoid cartilage at C6.

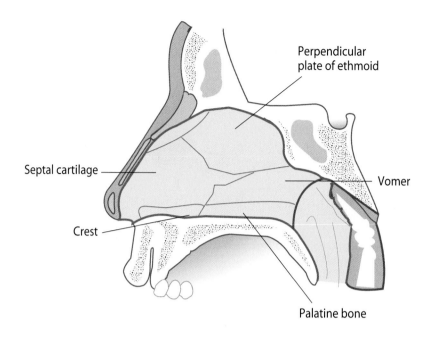

Figure 1.9. The skeleton of the nasal septum.

bony projections: the inferior, middle and superior turbinates (Figure 1.10). These vascular structures become engorged ipsilaterally, increasing airway resistance and reducing airflow, while those of the contralateral cavity contract. This normal alternating physiological process, the nasal cycle, may be more noticeable in patients with a septal deviation or in those with rhinitis.

The nasal cavity has an enormously rich blood supply, which originates from both the internal and external carotid arteries (Figure 1.11). As a result, epistaxis may result in considerable blood loss, resulting in death. In cases of intractable posterior nasal bleeding, the sphenopalatine artery may be endoscopically ligated by raising a mucoperiosteal flap on the lateral nasal wall. Bleeding from the ethmoidal vessels requires a periorbital incision and identification of these vessels as they pass from the orbital cavity into the nasal cavity in the fronto-ethmoidal suture.

The olfactory mucosa is limited to the roof and superior surface of the lateral wall of the nasal cavity (Figure 1.10). Olfactants, once dissolved in mucus, combine with olfactory binding proteins, which in turn bind to specific olfactory bipolar cells. Their axons converge to produce 12–20 olfactory bundles, which relay information superiorly to secondary neurones within the olfactory bulbs that lie over the cribiform fossae of the anterior cranial fossa.

The paranasal sinuses are paired, air-filled spaces that communicate with the nasal cavity via ostia located on the lateral nasal wall (Figure 1.12). Development of the paranasal sinuses occurs at different ages, although the frontal sinuses may not develop in a minority of patients.

Mucus produced by the respiratory epithelium within the paranasal sinuses does not drain entirely by gravity. In the maxillary sinus, for example, cilliary activity results in a spiral flow that directs mucus up and medially to the ostium high on the medial wall.

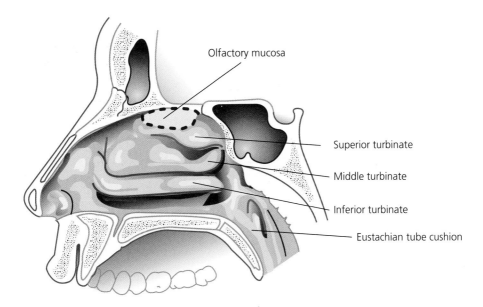

Figure 1.10. The lateral surface of the nasal cavity.

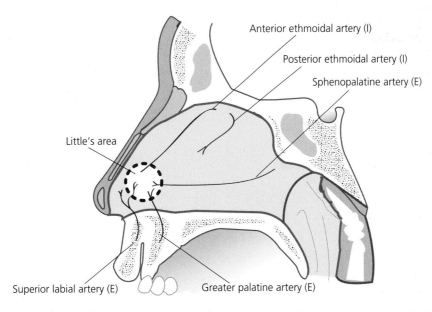

Figure 1.11. Arterial blood supply to the nose. The nose has a rich blood supply, supplied by both internal (I) and external (E) carotid arteries.

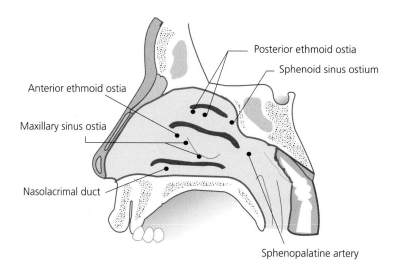

Figure 1.12. The lateral wall of the nasal cavity. (The turbinates have been removed in order to allow visualization of the ostia of the paranasal sinuses.)

The anterior and posterior ethmoidal air cells are separated from the orbital contents by the lamina papyracea, a thin plate of bone derived from the ethmoid bone. Infection within these paranasal sinuses may extend laterally, resulting in a subperiosteal abscess or orbital abscess, with eventual loss of vision. Extension posteriorly via the ophthalmic veins may result in cavernous sinus thrombosis and death.

The osteomeatal complex represents a region through which the paranasal sinuses drain (Figure 1.13). Obstruction may lead to acute or chronic sinusitis; hence opening this area is pivotal when surgically treating sinus disease.

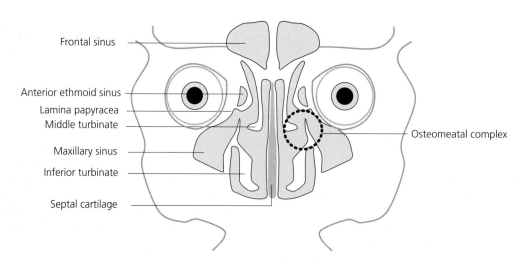

Figure 1.13. Coronal section of the paranasal sinuses.

ORAL CAVITY

The oral cavity is bounded anteriorly by the lips, posteriorly by the anterior tonsillar pillars, inferiorly by the tongue base and superiorly by the hard and soft palates (Figure 1.14).

The surface of the tongue is coarse, consisting of filliform and fungiform papillae.

The tongue is derived from mesoderm from the third and fourth branchial arches.

The sensory nerve supply to the surface of the tongue reflects its embryological development, the anterior two-thirds supplied by the mandibular division of the trigeminal nerve via the lingual nerve, the posterior third by the glossopharyngeal and superior laryngeal nerves.

The chorda tympani nerve, whose fibres hitchhike with the lingual nerve, supplies taste sensation to the anterior two-thirds of the tongue. Sweet, sour,

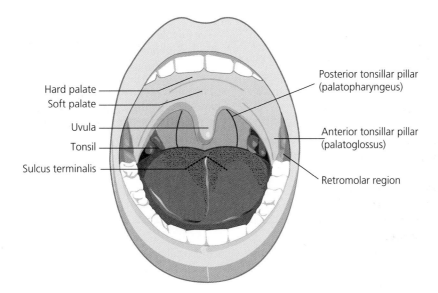

Figure 1.14. The oral cavity. The sulcus terminalis consists of the circumvallate papillae and represents the V-shaped junction of the anterior two-thirds and posterior third of the tongue. The foramen caecum, from which the thyroid gland originates, lies at the apex of the 'V'.

bitter and saltiness are detected by the fungiform papillae scattered along the superior margin of the tongue, and the filiform papillae.

The circumvallate papillae form an inverted 'V' that separates the anterior and posterior two-thirds of the tongue. The foramen caecum lies at the apex of this 'V' and represents the embryological site of origin of the thyroid gland. Rarely, due to failure of migration, a lingual thyroid may present as a mass at this site.

The tongue consists of a considerable mass of striated muscle separated in the midline by a fibrous membrane. Both intrinsic muscles (contained entirely within the tongue) and extrinsic muscles (inserted into bone) are supplied by the hypoglossal nerve, except for the palatoglossus (supplied by the pharyngeal plexus). A unilateral hypoglossal nerve palsy results in deviation of the tongue towards the side of the weakness.

The floor of the mouth is separated from the neck by the mylohyoid muscle. The muscle fans out from the lateral border of the hyoid bone to insert into the medial surface of the mandible as far back as the second molar tooth. A dental root infection that is anterior to this may result in an abscess forming in the floor of the mouth (Ludwig's angina). This is a potentially life-threatening airway emergency and requires urgent intervention to extract the affected tooth and drain the abscess.

The hyoid bone lies at the level of the third cervical vertebra. The larynx is suspended from this C-shaped bone and hence rises with the laryngeal skeleton during swallowing.

THE PHARYNX

The pharynx essentially consists of a fibrous cup, the pharyngobasilar fascia enclosed within a further three stacked muscular cups: the superior, middle and inferior constrictors. The muscle fibres of the constrictors sweep posteriorly and medially to meet in a midline posterior raphe. The pharyngeal plexus provides the motor supply to the musculature of the pharynx, except for stylopharyngeus, which is supplied by the glossopharyngeal nerve.

The superior constrictor arises from the medial pterygoid plate, hamulus, pterygomandibluar raphe and mandible. The Eustachian tube passes between its superior border and the skull base. Stylopharyngeus and the glossopharyngeal and lingual nerves pass below the constrictor.

The middle constrictor arises from the greater horn of the hyoid bone, its fibres sweeping to enclose the superior constrictor, and passing as low as the vocal cords.

The inferior constrictor consists of two striated muscles, the thyropharyngeus and cricopharyngeus. A potential area of weakness lies between the two muscles posteriorly: Killian's dehiscence. A posterior pulsion divertivulum may form a pharyngeal pouch within which food and debris may lodge.

THE NASOPHARYNX

The postnasal space, or nasopharynx, communicates with the middle ear cleft via the Eustachian tube (Figure 1.15). This tube opens during yawning and swallowing to allow air to pass into the middle ear cleft to maintain atmospheric pressure within the middle ear. This mechanism depends on

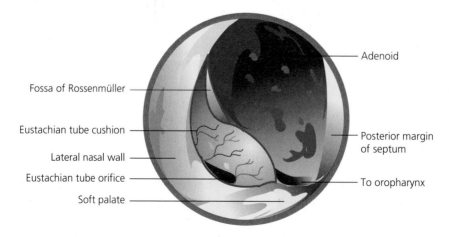

Adenoid

Fossa of Rossenmüller

Eustachian tube cushion

Lateral nasal wall

Eustachian tube orifice

Soft palate

Posterior margin of septum

To oropharynx

Figure 1.15. Endoscopic view of the right postnasal space.

normal soft palate musculature and hence a cleft palate is associated with chronic Eustachian tube dysfunction.

Blockage of the Eustachian tube may result in a middle ear effusion. This can be unilateral if due to a nasopharyngeal carcinoma arising from the fossa of Rossenmüller. An enlarged adenoidal pad may result in obstructive sleep apnoea, requiring surgical removal.

THE LARYNX

The principal function of the larynx is as a protective sphincter preventing aspiration of ingested material (Figure 1.16). Phonation is a secondary function. The three single cartilages of the larynx are the epiglottic, thyroid and cricoid cartilages. The three paired cartilages of the larynx are the arytenoid, corniculate and cuneiform cartilages.

The arytenoid cartilages are pyramidal structures from which the vocal cords project forward and medially. Abduction (lateral movement) of the cords is dependent on the posterior cricoarytenoid muscle, hence this is described as the most important muscle of the larynx. Additional instrinsic and extrinsic muscles provide adduction and variable cord tension.

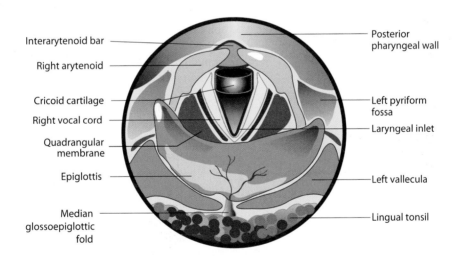

Figure 1.16. Endoscopic view of the larynx.

The motor supply of the muscles of the larynx is derived from the recurrent laryngeal nerves. An ipsilateral palsy results in hoarseness, while a bilateral palsy results in stridor and airway obstruction.

The cricoid is a signet ring-shaped structure which supports the arytenoid cartilages. As the only complete ring of cartilage in the airway, trauma may cause oedema and obstruction of the central lumen.

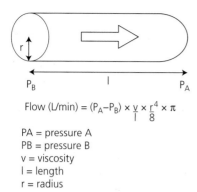

$$\text{Flow (L/min)} = (P_A - P_B) \times \frac{v}{l} \times \frac{r^4}{8} \times \pi$$

PA = pressure A
PB = pressure B
v = viscosity
l = length
r = radius

The Pouiseille-Hagan formula describes airflow through the lumen of a tube.

Reducing the lumen of a tube by half causes the flow to fall to 1/16th of the original. Therefore, trauma to the cricoid cartilage and oedema partially narrowing the lumen may result in a dramatic reduction in airflow.

THE MAJOR SALIVARY GLANDS

Whilst minor salivary glands are scattered within the oral cavity, saliva is predominantly produced by three paired major salivary glands: the parotid, submandibular and sublingual glands (Figure 1.17).

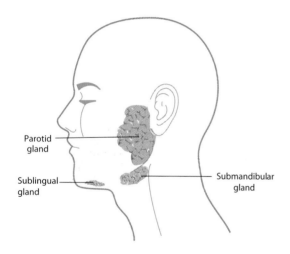

Parotid gland

Sublingual gland

Submandibular gland

Figure 1.17. The major salivary glands of the head and neck.

The parotid gland is a large, serous salivary gland enclosed by an extension of the investing layer of deep fascia of the neck. This parotid fascia is unforgiving and inflammation of the gland may result in severe pain.

Saliva produced by the parotid gland drains via Stenson's duct. The duct is approximately 5 cm in length and lies superficial to the masseter muscle. At the anterior border of this muscle it pierces the fibres of buccinator to enter the oral cavity opposite the upper 2nd molar tooth.

The facial nerve passes into and divides within the substance of the parotid gland to separate it into superficial and deep portions. Hence, an abscess or malignant lesion within the parotid gland may result in facial paralysis.

In addition, the retromandibular vein passes through the anterior portion of the gland and is a useful radiological marker for defining the superficial and deep portions of the gland.

The submandibular gland is a mixed serous and mucous salivary gland and forms the majority of saliva production at rest. Its superficial portion fills the space between the mandible and mylohyoid muscle, while its deep part lies between the mylohyoid and hyoglossus. The gland drains into the floor of the oral cavity via Wharton's duct, the papilla lying adjacent to the lingual frenulum. The duct may become obstructed by a calculus, which causes painful enlargement of the gland.

The sublingual glands lie anterior to hyoglossus in the sublingual fossa of the mandible. These mucus glands drain via multiple openings into the submandibular duct and sublingual fold in the floor of the oral cavity.

CERVICAL LYMPH NODES

The neck is divided into six levels. These describe groups of lymph nodes. Their landmarks are:

Level 1 – Submental and submandibular triangles, bounded by the midline, digastric and the mandible.

Level 2 – Anterior triangle including sternocleido-mastoid from skull base to the inferior border of hyoid.

Level 3 – Anterior triangle including sternocleido-mastoid from inferior border of hyoid to inferior border of cricoid.

Level 4 – Anterior triangle including sternoclei-domastoid from inferior border of cricoid to superior border of clavicle.

Level 5 – Posterior triangle: lateral border of sternocleidomastoid (SCM), superior border of clavicle, medial border of trapezius.

Level 6 – Paratracheal lymph nodes medial to the carotid.

These levels allow description of the various types of neck dissection that are performed when managing malignant disease (Figure 1.18). For example, a modified radical neck dissection involves removal of levels 1–5.

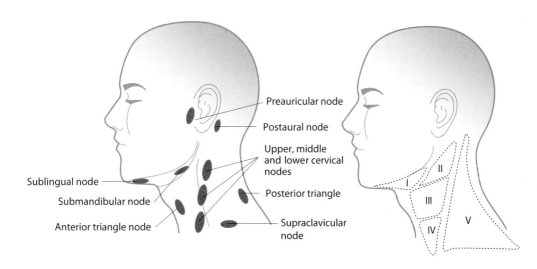

Figure 1.18. Lymph nodes groups and the triangles of the neck.

SENSORY DISTRIBUTION OF THE FACE

The sensory nerve supply of the face is derived from branches of the trigeminal nerve (Figure 1.19). Herpes zoster reactivation (shingles) will result in a pattern of vesicular eruption consistent with the distribution of that division.

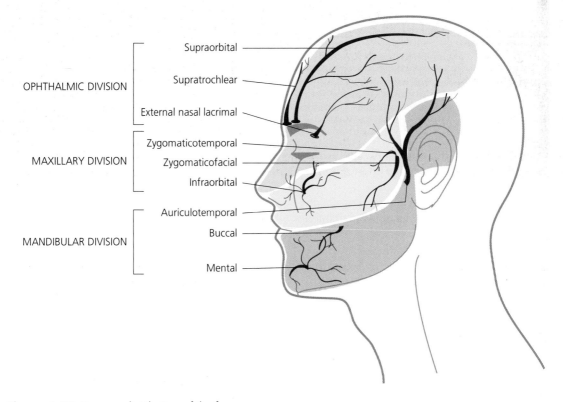

Figure 1.19. Sensory distribution of the face.

2 ENT EXAMINATION

A thorough clinical examination is essential in the diagnosis and management of any patient. This chapter provides a systematic and thorough, step-wise guide for clinicians assessing patients.

OTOSCOPY

Ensure that both you and the patient are seated comfortably and at the same level.

Examine the pinna, postaural region and adjacent scalp for scars, discharge, swelling and any skin lesions or defects (Figure 2.1). Choose the largest speculum that will fit comfortably into the ear and place it onto the otoscope.

Gently pull the pinna upwards and backwards to straighten the ear canal (backwards in children). Infection or inflammation may cause this manoeuvre to be painful.

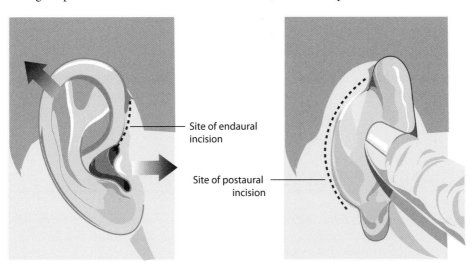

Site of endaural incision

Site of postaural incision

Figure 2.1. Examination of the pinna and postaural region. The pinna is pulled up and back and the tragus pushed forward in order to straighten the external auditory canal during otoscopy.

Hold the otoscope like a pen and rest your small digit on the patient's zygomatic arch. Any unexpected head movement will now push the speculum away from the ear, preventing trauma. Use the light to observe the direction of the ear canal and the tympanic membrane. The eardrum is better visualized by using the left hand for the left ear and the right hand for the right ear. Insert the speculum gently into the meatus, pushing the tragus forward. This further straightens the ear canal.

Inspect the entrance of the canal as you insert the speculum. Pass the tip through the hairs of the canal but no further. Looking through the otoscope, examine the ear canal and tympanic membrane (Figure 2.2). Adjust your position and the otoscope to view all of the tympanic membrane in a systematic manner. The ear cannot be judged to be normal until all areas of the tympanic membrane are viewed: the handle of malleus, pars tensa, pars flaccida (or attic) and anterior recess. If the view of the tympanic membrane is obscured by the presence of wax, this must be removed. If the patient has undergone mastoid surgery where the posterior ear canal wall has been removed, methodically inspect all parts of the cavity and tympanic membrane or drum remnant by adjusting your position. The normal appearance of a mastoid cavity varies, practice and experience will allow you to recognize pathology.

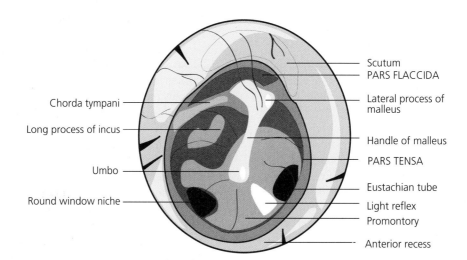

Figure 2.2. Examination of the right pinna. The scutum ('shield') is a thin plate of bone that obscures the view of the heads of the malleus and incus. It may be eroded by cholesteatoma and hence this area must always be inspected.

RINNE'S AND WEBER'S TUNING FORK TESTING

Although there have been various reports regarding the reliability of tuning fork tests (1), they are simple, quick and invaluable aids in the diagnosis of hearing loss (2). Tuning fork tests can be used to confirm audiometric findings, especially if the hearing test does not seem to be congruent with the clinical findings. They are also useful as a quick bedside test for checking that the patient has not suffered a dead ear following surgery.

Traditionally, a 512 Hz tuning fork is used for testing. Low-frequency tuning forks provide greater vibrotactile stimulation (which can be misinterpreted as an audible signal by the patient), while high-frequency tuning forks have a higher rate of decay (i.e., the tone does not last long after the tuning fork has been struck). There is evidence to suggest, however, that a 256 Hz tuning fork is more reliable than a 512 Hz tuning fork (3,4).

The commonest tuning fork tests performed are the Rinne's and Weber's tests. They must be performed in conjunction in order to diagnose a conductive or sensorineural hearing loss.

Rinne's test

A 512 Hz tuning fork is struck on the elbow. It is essential that the examiner checks that they can hear the tuning fork as this also serves as a comparative test of hearing. The tuning fork is presented to the patient with the prongs of the fork held vertically and in line with the ear canal. The patient is asked if they can hear a sound. The tuning fork is held by the ear for a few moments before its base is firmly pressed against the mastoid process behind the ear. The patient is asked, 'Is it louder in front or when I place it on your head?'

As air conduction (AC) is better that bone conduction (BC) in a normal hearing ear, the tuning fork is heard louder in front of the ear than when placed behind the ear (i.e., AC > BC). This is described as Rinne +ve; if bone conduction is greater than air conduction, this is Rinne −ve.

Weber's test

A 512 Hz tuning fork is struck on the elbow and firmly placed on the patient's forehead. The patient is asked, 'Is the sound louder in your left ear, right ear, or somewhere in the middle?'

As the hearing in both ears should be the same, in a normal subject the sound heard will be 'in the middle'.

Interpretation

In order to diagnose a conductive or sensorineural hearing loss, both Rinne's and Weber's tests must be performed (Figure 2.3).

If Rinne's test is +ve on the left and −ve on the right, and Weber's test lateralizes to the right side, this suggests a conductive hearing loss in the right ear.

If Rinne's test is −ve on the right and +ve on the left, and Weber's test lateralizes to the left side, this suggests a right sensorineural hearing loss in the right ear.

Anterior rhinoscopy

The head mirror is often approached with some trepidation by the junior ENT surgeon, who may feel self-conscious as the mirror can be cumbersome. Many departments use headlights as an alternative.

A right-handed examiner should position the Bull's lamp over the patient's left shoulder at head height and wear the head mirror over their right eye. The lamp light can be directed onto the head mirror and the beam focused onto the patient.

Examine the profile of the nose, looking for external deviation of the nasal dorsum. Check for bruising, swelling, signs of infection, nasal discharge and scars.

Gently raise the tip of the nose to allow you to examine the vestibule of the nose and the antero-inferior end of the nasal septum.

The Thudichum speculum is held in the non-dominant hand (i.e., the left if the examiner is right-handed), leaving the dominant hand free to use any instruments.

Hold the metal loop on your index finger with the finger pointing towards you and the prongs away from you.

Swing your middle finger to one side of the Thudichum and your ring finger to the other. You can now squeeze the Thudichum and use the prongs to open the nares to examine the nasal cavity. This provides a view of the nasal septum, inferior turbinate and head of the middle turbinate. A flexible nasolaryngoscope or a rigid endoscope is required

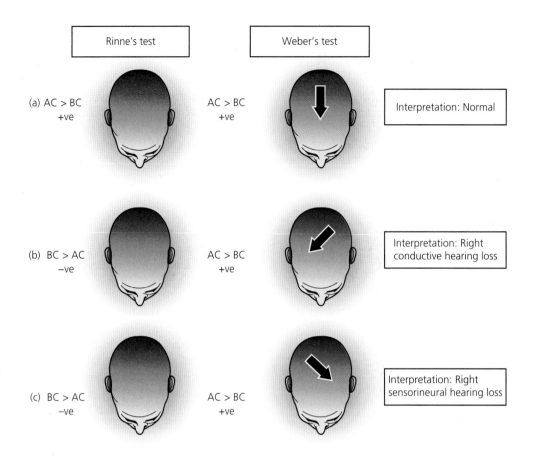

Rinne's test	Weber's test

(a) AC > BC
+ve

AC > BC
+ve

Interpretation: Normal

(b) BC > AC
−ve

AC > BC
+ve

Interpretation: Right conductive hearing loss

(c) BC > AC
−ve

AC > BC
+ve

Interpretation: Right sensorineural hearing loss

Figure 2.3. Interpretation of tuning fork tests.

in order to assess the middle meatus, posterior nasal cavity and postnasal space.

In children, especially if a foreign body is suspected, it is often kinder simply to lift the tip of the nose rather than use a Thudichum speculum. Alternatively, an otoscope provides an excellent view.

Nasal patency is assessed by placing a metal speculum under the nose. Misting or condensation on the metal surface during expiration provides a measure of nasal patency.

▌ Ear microsuction

Explain to the patient that microsuction is required in order to remove debris and wax from the external auditory canal. Warn the patient that they will hear a loud hissing noise and may experience temporary dizziness following the procedure.

Position the patient supine (or sitting in a chair) with the head turned to the opposite side. With the microscope illuminating the ear, take this opportunity to study the pinna, canal opening and surrounding skin for scars or sinuses.

Adjust the eye pieces and start with the lowest magnification. Use the largest speculum that will comfortably enter the external auditory canal. Hold the speculum between the index finger and thumb, place the middle finger into the conchal bowl and gently pull the pinna posteriorly. This will open and straighten the ear canal. If the ear canal is narrow, use a smaller speculum or ask the patient to open their mouth (this manoeuvre often increases the antero-posterior diameter of the canal as the condyl of the mandible is related to the anterior canal wall).

Assess the canal wall and contents. Remember that the hairy outer third of the canal is relatively insensitive but the thin inner skin is exquisitely sensitive. Any contact with the speculum or suction will produce a great deal of discomfort.

Using a wide bore sucker, begin by removing debris within the lateral hairy portion of the canal. Aim to touch only the debris and not the canal skin. Try to remove all the debris, especially in cases of otitis externa where debris will result in ongoing infection if not removed. A wax hook may be used as an alternative method for wax removal.

If the debris or wax is too hard or the procedure too uncomfortable for the patient, a course of sodium bicarbonate ear drops (two drops three times a day for two weeks) will be required before a further attempt at wax removal is made.

If the tympanic membrane is obscured, microsuction along the anterior canal wall until the tympanic membrane is visible (the tympanic membrane is continuous with the posterior canal wall and can be damaged if microsuction follows the posterior canal wall).

If there is trauma to the ear canal or if bleeding occurs, prescribe a short course of antibiotic ear drops, warning the patient of the risk of ototoxicity.

▮ Flexible nasolaryngoscopy

Explain the procedure to the patient and ask the patient which side of their nose is the easier to breathe through, selecting this side for examination. Spray the chosen side with local anaesthetic or insert a cotton wool pledget soaked in local anaesthetic. Patients often describe numbness of the upper lip or back of their tongue, which can be used as a guide to the level of anaesthesia.

The nasoendoscope may be used with or without a sheath, depending on local decontamination protocols. Clean the tip of the scope with an alcohol wipe to prevent condensation and apply a thin film of lubricant gel to the distal 5 cm of the nasoendoscope. Ensure the gel does not cover the tip of the scope as this will occlude your view. The patient's saliva provides an effective alternative.

Ask the patient to breathe through their mouth and, holding the end of the scope between the index finger and thumb, place the tip of the nasoendoscope into the nasal cavity. Ensure full control of the scope by placing the middle finger on the tip of the patient's nose. If a patient were to fall forward, the nasoendoscope will not be driven into the nasal cavity.

Insert the scope into the nostril and pass it along the floor of the nose with the inferior turbinate laterally and septum medially. Posteriorly, the Eustachian tube orifice and postnasal space will come into view (see Chapter 1, Figure 1.2). If the septum is deviated and the scope cannot be easily advanced, try to pass it between the inferior and middle turbinates (laterally) and the septum (medially). If this is too uncomfortable for the patient, the other nasal cavity may be used.

With the postnasal space in view, ask the patient to breathe in through their nose. This opens the inlet into the oropharynx. Use the control toggle to flex the distal end of the scope inferiorly and gently advance.

The uvula and soft palate will slide away and the base of tongue and larynx will come into view (see Chapter 1, Figure 1.14).

Adopt a system to ensure that all aspects of this region are examined. The following is a guide: tongue base, valleculae, epiglottis (lingual and laryngeal surfaces), supraglottis, interarytenoid bar, vocal cords (appearance and mobility), subglottis, pyriform fossae and posterior pharyngeal wall. The larynx may be difficult to view in those patients with an infantile epiglottis or prominent tongue base. Where this is encountered, ask the patient to point their chin up to the ceiling to draw the tongue base forward and bring the larynx into view. To assess the pyriform fossae, ask the patient to blow their cheeks out while you pinch their nose. If secretions obscure your view, ask the patient to swallow.

Remove the scope gently and supply patients with tissues to use after completing the examination.

▌ Rigid nasoendoscopy

Rigid endoscopy of the nasal cavity requires a systematic examination involving three passes with either a 0° or 30° scope (Figure 2.4).

The first pass provides an overall view of the anterior nasal cavity, the septum and the floor

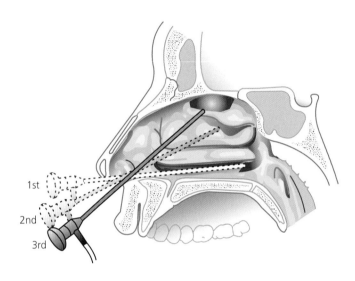

Figure 2.4. Rigid endoscopy. The first pass of the endoscope should pass along the floor of the nose, the second is into the middle meatus and the third into the superior meatus and olfactory niche.

of the nasal cavity to the posterior choana. The Eustachian tube cushion, orifice and the fossa of Rossenmüller, and adenoidal pad must also be examined.

The second is into the middle meatus and allows identification of the uncinate process, middle meatal ostium and ethmoidal bulla. The third examines the superior meatus and olfactory niche; the sphenoid ostium may be identified during this pass.

▌ Examination of the oral cavity

Ensure that both you and the patient are seated comfortably, at the same level.

Using the head mirror or headlight, begin by examining the lips and face of the patient. Note any scars or petechiae.

It is important to be systematic (Figure 2.5). Use two tongue depressors. Begin by asking the patient to open their mouth and insert one tongue depressor onto the buccal surface of each cheek and ask the patient to clench their teeth. Gently pulling laterally, withdraw the blades examining the buccal mucosa, gingivae, teeth, parotid duct orifices and buccal sulci. Anteriorly, draw the blades superiorly to examine beneath the upper lip and repeat with the lower lip.

Ask the patient to open their mouth and study the superior surface of the tongue. With the tongue

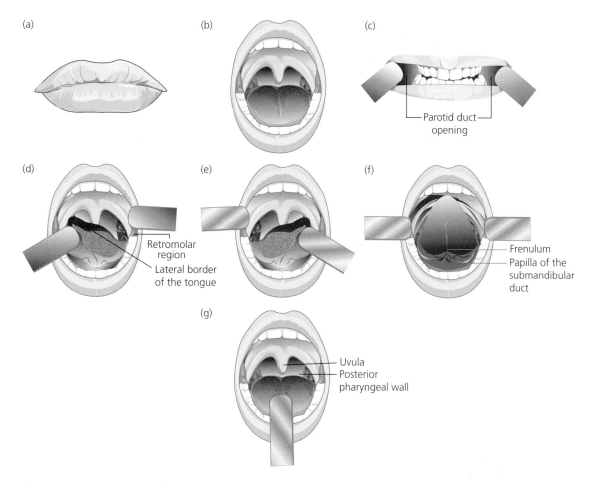

(a)

(b)

(c)
Parotid duct opening

(d)
Retromolar region
Lateral border of the tongue

(e)

(f)
Frenulum
Papilla of the submandibular duct

(g)
Uvula
Posterior pharyngeal wall

Figure 2.5. Examination of the oral cavity. A systematic approach must be used to assess the oral cavity fully.

pointing superiorly, examine the floor of the mouth and inferior surface of the tongue. The openings of the submandibular ducts are found just lateral to the frenulum of the tongue.

Using both tongue blades again, examine the retromolar regions and lateral borders of the tongue.

Ask the patient to keep their tongue in their mouth and keep breathing. Gently depress the anterior half of the tongue, avoiding the posterior third as this can make patients gag. Examine both tonsils, comparing their relative size. Inspect the oropharynx, including uvula and movements of the soft palate. Ask the patient to look up to the ceiling and examine the hard palate.

Palpate the tongue including the tongue base. Submucosal tumours in these structures can often be palpated before they are seen. Where the history is suggestive of an abnormality of the submandibular gland or duct, bimanual palpation should be used.

▌ Examination of the neck and facial nerve function

Inspect the general appearance of the patient, noting any facial scars or asymmetry of facial tone at rest. Ensure adequate exposure of the patient by removing neck ties and unfasten the upper shirt buttons so that both clavicles are visualized.

Inspect the neck, noting scars, sinuses, masses or tattoos (these were previously used to mark radiotherapy fields).

Stand behind the subject and sequentially palpate the same lymph node levels on both sides of the neck simultaneously (Figure 2.5). It is important to be systematic. Start with the submental then submandibular triangles (level 1), followed by the jugulodigastric and jugular lymph nodes (levels 2, 3, 4) by palpating along the anterior border of each sternocleidomastoid muscle and the paratracheal region. Examine the posterior triangle nodes. Working posteriorly, palpate the parotid gland, postaural and occipital lymph nodes.

Once again, palpate the laryngeal skeleton and thyroid gland from behind. Note the site, size and appearance of any mass and whether it is tethered to the skin or underlying muscles. Assess whether the mass moves with swallowing (give the patient a glass of water to drink) or tongue protrusion. Auscultate for a bruit and, in the case of a thyroid mass with retrosternal extension, percuss from superior to inferior along the sternum.

▋ Examination of facial nerve function

Sitting level with the patient, examine their general appearance and for any scars or masses.

Ask the patient to raise their eyebrows and compare both sides. Remember that there is crossover in the innervation of this region so that a patient is still able to wrinkle their forehead in a unilateral upper motor neuron palsy.

Ask the patient to shut their eyes tightly, flare their nostrils, blow out their cheeks and bare their teeth. Where facial weakness is observed, blinking repeatedly may reveal synkinesis where reinnervation has occurred along incorrect pathways; contraction of obicularis oris may result in contraction of the angle of the mouth.

All patients must have their facial weakness graded so that any changes can be monitored.

The most commonly used grading system is the House-Brackmann facial grading system. Note that there is complete eye closure in a grade 3 and incomplete eye closure in a grade 4 facial palsy.

Grade 1 – Normal.
Grade 2 – Slight weakness with good eye closure with minimal effort, good forehead movement and slight asymmetry of the mouth.
Grade 3 – Symmetry and normal tone at rest with obvious weakness, although complete eye closure and asymmetrical mouth movement with effort.
Grade 4 – Incomplete eye closure, no movement of the forehead, but symmetry and normal tone at rest.
Grade 5 – Asymmetry at rest with barely perceptible movement of the mouth and incomplete eye closure.
Grade 6 – No movement.

When faced with a true lower motor neuron palsy, look for a cause by examining the remaining cranial nerves, perform otoscopy to exclude middle ear pathology and palpate the parotid glands. Audiology is required with tympanometry, a pure tone audiogram and occasionally stapedial reflexes.

REFERENCES

1 Burkey JM, Lippy WH, Schuring AG, Rizer FM (1998). Clinical utility of the 512-Hz Rinne tuning fork test. *Am J Otol* **19**: 59–62.
2 Behn A, Westerberg BD, Zhang H, *et al* (2007). Accuracy of the Weber and Rinne tuning fork tests in evaluation of children with otitis media with effusion. *J Otolaryngol* **36**: 197–202.
3 Browning GG, Swan IR (1988). Sensitivity and specificity of Rinne tuning fork test. *BMJ* **297**: 1381–2.
4 Browning GG, Swan IR, Chew KK (1989). Clinical role of informal tests of hearing. *J Laryngol Otol* **103**: 7–11.

3

COMMON ENT PATHOLOGY

OTITIS EXTERNA

Otitis externa is inflammation of the external auditory canal. It is common, extremely painful and often precipitated by irritants such as cotton buds. There may be an infective component, commonly bacterial, such as *Pseudomonas aeruginosa*, *Staphylococcus aureus* and *Proteus*, or less frequently fungal, such as *Aspergillus* species or *Candida albicans*. The external auditory canal is often swollen and filled with debris, that requires microsuction. Treatment is with one week of ear drops containing a combination of steroid and antibiotic. Fungal infections require a 3–4-week course of anti-fungal drops. An ear swab is useful in directing antibiotic selection where the infection does not resolve with the initial treatment.

When the external ear canal is very swollen, a wick is inserted to splint the meatus open to allow penetration of the topical treatment. This should be removed as the swelling decreases, usually after 48 hours. The infection may progress to involve the pinna and peri-auricular soft tissues (cellulitis), necessitating hospital admission for intravenous antibiotics. Sometimes the infection is localized and a small abscess, or furuncle, can form. This is

commonly caused by *S. aureus* infection of a hair follicle in the ear canal and is exquisitely painful. Incision and drainage are often required, together with topical antibiotics.

An important differential diagnosis of otitis externa is malignant otitis externa, which is a necrotizing osteomyelitis of the ear canal and lateral skull base, which occurs more frequently in diabetics and immunocompromised patients. *Pseudomonas aeruginosa* is the most common cause and the typical otoscopic appearance is granulation tissue or exposed bone on the floor of the ear canal. As the infection spreads through the skull base, the lower cranial nerves (CN VII–XII) are affected. The diagnosis is usually made on computerized tomography (CT) scan and the treatment is a prolonged (six-week) course of intravenous antibiotics followed by further oral antibiotics, regular microsuction, topical antibiotic–steroid ear drops, good glycaemic control and analgesia. Sometimes a biopsy is needed to exclude malignancy and determine microbiological sensitivities. Radioisotope scans (e.g., gallium) or magnetic resonance imaging (MRI) can be used to assess the response to treatment.

IMPACTED WAX

Ear wax is composed of secretions from sebaceous and apocrine glands in the lateral third of the ear canal mixed with dead squamous cells. It becomes

impacted in 10% of children, 5% of healthy adults and nearly 60% of the elderly (1). Although often asymptomatic, it may cause a significant conductive hearing loss and discomfort. Impacted wax needs to be removed to facilitate examination of the tympanic membrane. In primary care, removal is facilitated by the use of ceruminolytic agents (2) or ear syringing. Syringing is, however, contraindicated in those who have a tympanic membrane perforation or who have developed otitis externa following previous syringing. In otolaryngology departments, wax is removed under the microscope using a Zoellner sucker, wax hook, Jobson-Horne probe or crocodile forceps. Care should be taken to avoid trauma to the ear canal. The use of cotton buds by the patient should be discouraged as this impacts the wax and traumatises the ear canal causing otitis externa.

ACUTE OTITIS MEDIA (AOM)

Inflammation of middle ear mucosa mainly affects young children as part of an upper respiratory tract infection. Causative organisms include viruses and bacteria, such as *Streptococcus pneumoniae*, *Haemophilus influenza* and *Moraxella catarrhalis*. Patients present with general symptoms of irritability, pyrexia and nausea, with ENT symptoms of otalgia and hearing loss. Examination reveals a bulging erythematous tympanic membrane, which may perforate and discharge pus. Initial treatment is supportive, with simple analgesia or antipyretics. If symptoms persist, oral antibiotics such as amoxicillin or clarithromycin are indicated (3). Frequent episodes of AOM (more than four episodes over six months) require ENT referral. Recurrent otitis media may be treated by insertion of grommets or long-term antibiotics.

Rare but potentially serious complications of AOM (and more commonly of acute mastoiditis – see below) can be classified anatomically into three groups:

1 Intratemporal – Tympanic membrane perforation, facial nerve palsy (particularly if the tympanic segment of facial nerve is dehiscent) and acute mastoiditis with mastoid abscess.
2 Intracranial – Meningitis, brain abscess, encephalitis and sigmoid sinus thrombosis.
3 Systemic – Septicaemia, septic arthritis and endocarditis.

OTITIS MEDIA WITH EFFUSION (OME) (GLUE EAR)

Persistent otitis media with bilateral effusions (OME) is the most common cause of hearing loss in children. The typical audiological finding is a mild to moderate conductive hearing loss, associated with a flat (type B) tympanogram. Bilateral grommet insertion is indicated (4) where effusions persist for over three months associated with a hearing level in the better hearing ear of 25–30 dB HL or worse, averaged at 0.5, 1, 2 and 4 kHz. Children with Down's syndrome should be offered hearing aids rather than grommet surgery if they have OME. Children with cleft palate can be offered grommets as an alternative to hearing aids.

Adults with persistent unilateral OME should undergo examination of the postnasal space under general anaesthesia, with a biopsy taken from the fossa of Rosenmüller, immediately posterior to the Eustachian tube orifice, to exclude the possibility of a nasopharyngeal tumour.

ACUTE MASTOIDITIS

Acute mastoiditis is an inflammatory process affecting the mastoid air cells; it occurs most commonly in children. It is an uncommon complication of acute otitis media. Patients are generally unwell, with spiking temperatures. There is a post-auricular abscess with lateral and anterior displacement of the pinna and tenderness over the mastoid bone. The majority of cases respond to medical treatment with intravenous antibiotics, analgesia and hydration (5). A contrast-enhanced CT scan is used to exclude a brain abscess, lateral sinus thrombosis and assess temporal bone anatomy, particularly where there is failure to improve after 48 hours or the suspicion of complications demands surgical intervention (see above); commonly, cortical mastoidectomy and grommet insertion with placement of a corrugated drain within the post-auricular wound.

PINNA HAEMATOMA

Blunt trauma to the pinna may result in a sub-periosteal haematoma. Since the cartilage gains its nutrient supply from the overlying perichondrium, an untreated pinna haematoma results in cartilage necrosis and permanent deformity – 'cauliflower ear'. Needle aspiration of a pinna haematoma followed by a compression bandage is rarely effective. A small incision through the overlying skin under local anaesthetic allows continued drainage and is a more definitive treatment (6). The incision should be placed where the scar will be least visible, ideally along the rim of the conchal bowl, under the helical rim or approached from the cranial surface of the pinna (with a small window of cartilage excised). 'Through-and-through' sutures can be placed to secure silastic splints or dental rolls, to achieve more reliable pressure and prevent haematoma recurrence under the head bandage. All patients should receive co-amoxiclav or an equivalent antibiotic to prevent perichondritis and be reviewed after 7 days for suture removal.

PERICHONDRITIS AND PINNA CELLULITIS

Inflammation of the perichondrium (perichondritis) can result in a permanent deformity of the pinna. It commonly occurs as a result of bacterial infection following trauma to the pinna from a piercing, insect bite or skin abrasion, although can also be secondary to otis externa. The pinna is swollen, erythematous and extremely tender. Previous episodes of perichondritis or inflammation of other cartilaginous structures should be sought in order to exclude relapsing perichondritis.

Perichondritis and pinna cellulitis require a combination of intravenous and oral antibiotics as cartilage compromise can lead to marked disfigurement of the pinna. Piercings in the affected ear should be removed. Rarely, surgery is required to drain a collection or debride necrotic soft tissue (7).

SUDDEN SENSORINEURAL HEARING LOSS (SSHL)

This is a unilateral or bilateral subjective deterioration in hearing, which develops over seconds to hours and on objective testing is confirmed to be sensorineural in nature. A conductive hearing loss should first be excluded by careful examination of the ear, tuning fork tests and a pure tone audiogram. In 88% of cases, no obvious cause is found, but a careful history and examination should consider potential infective, auto-immune, vascular, traumatic, neoplastic and neurological causes (8). Competing theories for idiopathic cases include viral and vascular insults to the inner ear and rupture of the cochlear membrane. Approximately 60% of patients improve with or without intervention and evidence for any particular treatment is mixed. Treatment options include prednisolone (oral or injected into the middle ear) (9), aspirin, betashistine (10), acyclovir and inhaled carbogen (oxygen mixed with 5% CO_2) (11). Unilateral loss may be managed in the outpatient setting, but those with bilateral loss require admission for investigation (blood tests to exclude autoimmune causes and MRI scanning).

FACIAL NERVE PALSY

There are a wide variety of causes for a facial nerve palsy. Lower motor neurone lesions are distinguished from upper motor neurone lesions by the absence of forehead movement (forehead movement is spared in upper motor neurone lesions as a result of the bilateral upper motor neurone distribution supplying this area). All patients must have their degree of facial weakness recorded using the House Brackmann scale.

Lower motor neurone pathology can occur anywhere along the path of the affected nerve. An assessment of the cranial nerves, ear, parotid gland, oral cavity and neck examination is mandatory.

Causes include Bell's palsy, Ramsay Hunt Syndrome, malignant otits externa, ear or parotid surgery, middle ear disease temporal bone fracture and iatrogenic trauma.

▮ Bells palsy

This syndrome of facial paralysis is a diagnosis of exclusion. Although described as idiopathic, there is evidence to suggest the palsy occurs due to herpes reactivation. A thorough history and examination are required. An MRI is only indicated if this is a recurrent palsy or if the palsy fails to recover (12).

Initial treatment is with oral prednisolone (1 mg per kg, typically 60 mg for an adult) for seven days. Although there is inconclusive evidence to support the use of antivirals, acyclovir (800 mg five times a day for 10 days) is also often prescribed (13). Any patient with a facial nerve palsy who is unable to close their eye (House-Brackmann grade 4–6) must use artificial tears and tape their eye closed at night in order to protect the cornea. If the eye becomes painful or red an urgent ophthalmic opinion should be sought.

Approximately 60% of patients with an idiopathic palsy recover to House Brackmann grade 1 or 2. A further 12% suffer a recurrence on the same or contralateral side.

▮ Ramsay Hunt syndrome

This condition is caused by herpes zoster. The facial palsy is accompanied by painful vesicles on the pinna or external auditory canal, and occasionally the soft palate. Onset is rapid and the 8th nerve may become involved with concurrent hearing loss and vertigo. Treatment is similar to that of Bell's palsy (14,15).

▮ Acute suppurative otitis media (ASOM)

An acute otitis media may result in a facial nerve palsy, typically if the bony canal of the facial nerve is dehiscent within the middle ear cleft. Treatment includes intravenous antibiotics, oral steroids and nasal decongestants. CT of the temporal bone may be of value in order to exclude chrinoc suppurative oititis media (CSOM). A myringotomy may be considered appropriate if there is no clinical improvement following 24–48 hours of medical treatment.

▮ Trauma

Every patient undergoing middle ear surgery must have their facial nerve function recorded pre- and post-operatively. Iatrogenic damage may require surgical re-exploration and nerve repair.

FOREIGN BODIES–EAR

Foreign bodies within the external ear canal commonly affect children and may be difficult to remove. Children will need to be held by a parent or nurse, and the first attempt at removal is often the only chance. If the foreign body cannot be removed, a short general anaesthetic in the following few days is indicated to allow removal. The exception are batteries, which are corrosive and must be removed that day. Objects can be removed under the microscope using a wax hook, microsuction or irrigation (Figure 3.1). The use of crocodile forceps can result in medial displacement of the foreign bodies and their use should be restricted to objects that can be grasped. Insects should be drowned using olive oil prior to removal. *Do not attempt to flush out tablets, seeds or nuts (organic materials) as these swell and become more difficult to remove.*

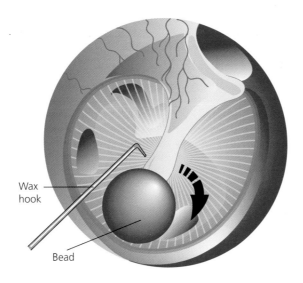

Wax hook

Bead

Figure 3.1. Removal of a bead from the external auditory canal.

TYMPANIC MEMBRANE TRAUMA

Pressure changes or direct trauma can damage the external auditory canal and tympanic membrane. On otoscopy, the tympanic membrane is often obscured by blood. Tuning fork tests and audiograms are used to assess hearing. Hearing loss may be conductive due to blood in the middle or external ear or ossicular discontinuity. Sensorineural hearing loss is more common when there is an accompanying temporal bone fracture.

Treatment is generally conservative. Patients are reassured and advised to keep the ear dry and have an outpatient follow-up at six weeks, where spontaneous healing of tympanic membrane is usually confirmed. An audiogram documents return of hearing to normal.

TEMPORAL BONE FRACTURES

The temporal bone contains many vital structures, including the facial nerve, cochlea, labyrinth, ossicles, internal carotid artery, jugular vein and sigmoid sinus. Temporal bone fractures are traditionally classified as longitudinal, transverse and oblique, in relation to the petrous ridge of the temporal bone. The usefulness of this classification system has been questioned and a newer system categorizing injuries on CT as otic-capsule violating and otic-capsule sparing has been shown to be more predictive of complications (16). Initially, advanced trauma life support (ATLS) management takes priority as temporal bone fractures can be associated with significant head injury. Clinical signs include blood in the ear canal, haemotympanum and Battle's sign (post-auricular bruising). Of more concern are sensorineural hearing loss, vertigo, facial nerve injury and cerebral spinal fluid (CSF) otorrhoea.

Facial nerve function immediately after injury must be documented. CT scanning is helpful in excluding intracranial injury, identifying damage to important intra-temporal structures and classifying the type of fracture. Immediate-onset severe facial nerve paralysis is suggestive of nerve transection and may require surgical exploration. However, most traumatic facial nerve palsies are delayed in onset, secondary to fracture-related nerve oedema and are treated conservatively with steroids.

FOREIGN BODIES–NOSE

Foreign bodies in the nose should be removed as soon as possible as there is a theoretical risk of aspiration (Figure 3.2). As with foreign bodies in the ear, children need to be held by a parent or nurse, often with a blanket wrapped around the body and arms. A headlight, suction and wax hook allow removal in most cases. A useful additional removal technique is the 'parent's kiss', whereby the parent blows air into the mouth of the child while occluding the contralateral nostril (17). If these manoeuvres are unsuccessful, a short general anaesthetic is required for removal.

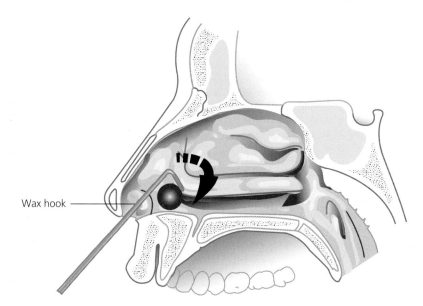

Wax hook

Figure 3.2. Removal of a foreign body from the nasal cavity.

NASAL TRAUMA

Nasal trauma may result in a deviated bridge. A patient who has sustained a nasal injury, with suspected deviation of the nasal bones should be first assessed for other injuries (ATLS protocol).

The nose should be examined to exclude a septal haematoma and any epistaxis managed. Swelling over the nose may prevent an accurate assessment of the position of the nasal bones. Hence, the patient should be recalled 5–7 days post injury and the nasal bridge reassessed.

If the nasal bones are deviated, and the patient desires it, the nose can be manipulated under local or general anaesthesia (18). It is essential that this is performed within 14 days of the initial injury as the bridge may become fixed, making simple manipulation impossible. Risks include epistaxis, periorbital bruising and septal haematoma. Patients should be warned that the aim is to straighten the bony bridge and that their nose may appear different to that

prior to the injury. The nose will remain unstable until the bones have re-healed and so further injury should be avoided.

SEPTAL HAEMATOMA / ABSCESS

Septal haematomas can rapidly develop following nasal trauma or after septal surgery. A haematoma can become secondarily infected resulting in an abscess. Patients describe nasal obstruction and pain. Examination usually reveals bilateral septal swelling, which is compressible on palpation. Pus may be seen lying on the surface of the septum.

Patients require formal incision and drainage under general anaesthetic. A hemitransfixtion incision is

made and a corrugated drain sutured in place (a trouser drain may be required with a 'leg' on either side of the septal cartilage). Antibiotic treatment is required following abscess drainage and a pus swab sent to microbiology. A septal haematoma or abscess should be seen within a few hours and operated on within a day, as prolonged devascularisation of the cartilage results in its re-absorption resulting in nasal deformity (19). In addition, infection may extend intracranially via the ophthalmic veins to involve the cavernous sinus.

ACUTE SINUSITIS

Acute sinusitis is generally managed in primary care with oral antibiotics and nasal decongestants. It commonly occurs following an acute upper respiratory tract infection and presents with purulent nasal discharge, nasal obstruction and facial pain that is

worse on bending forward. Patients may be referred if there are concerns regarding complications of sinusitis such as periorbital cellulitis. Fungal sinusitis should be considered when assessing patients who are immuno-compromised.

PERIORBITAL CELLULITIS

Periorbital cellulitis is an ENT emergency and patients may become blind within a matter of hours. A subperiosteal abscess may arise due to spread of infection from the ethmoidal air cells laterally into the orbital cavity. Patients often describe a recent upper respiratory tract infection. These patients must be discussed promptly with a senior colleague so that they can be reviewed or their management discussed.

The eyelids may be swollen with associated chemosis, and there may be proptosis of the eye. It is important to assess red colour vision, in particular, and this may be performed using an Ishihara chart. Visual acuity and eye movements, also require regular monitoring. Restricted eye movement or pain on eye movement is often associated with an abscess. Given that the condition predominantly occurs in children, such an examination can be challenging

and it is worth seeking paediatric and ophthalmological consultations early. Patients with periorbital cellulitis or a potential intraorbital collection should be discussed promptly with a senior so that they can be reviewed or their management discussed.

An urgent CT scan of the paranasal sinuses is essential. For young children preparations may be made to perform the scan under general anaesthetic, proceeding to surgery if the imaging reveals a collection. Children should receive appropriate analgesia, intravenous antibiotics (normally a 3rd generation cephalosporin) and, if there is evidence of sinusitis, paediatric nasal decongestant.

Surgical decompression of a subperiosteal abscess is performed endoscopically or via a Lynch-Howarth incision. A drain is required if an open approach is used.

TONSILLITIS

Tonsillitis is most commonly bacterial, caused by *Streptococci*, *Staphylococci* or *Haemophilus influenza*. Viral infections also occur, most commonly the *Epstein-Barr* virus (EBV), which is the cause of infectious mononucleosis or glandular fever. Patients have a painful throat with odynophagia (pain on swallowing) and sometimes referred otalgia. They are treated in primary care with phenoxymethylpenicillin (Penicillin V), or a macrolide if they are penicillin-allergic. Ampicillin, Amoxicillin and Co-Amoxiclav should be avoided as these can precipitate a severe scarring rash in patients with EBV.

If patients are unable to swallow fluids, they should be admitted to hospital for re-hydration and intravenous antibiotics. Bloods are sent for a full blood count, electrolytes, liver function tests, C reactive protein, and the locally-agreed test for EBV.

Intravenous benzylpenicillin is required and oral soluble paracetamol, codeine and a non-steroidal anti-inflammatory for analgesia. Tonsillar enlargement may cause airway obstruction, and if there is any suggestion of compromise patients must undergo flexible nasolaryngoscopy. In such cases, these patients should be given steroids (either 8 mg dexamethasone IV or hydrocortisone 200 mg IV), discussed with a senior colleague and closely monitored in an ENT airway observation bed or in a high dependency or critical care unit. If, conversely, a patient complains of a severe sore throat and has tonsils with *normal* appearances, immediate nasolaryngoscopy should be performed to assess whether the diagnosis is supraglottitis.

Inpatient treatment is normally required for no more than 24–48 hours and patients are discharged with analgesia and oral antibiotics. A short course of steroids may be useful in patients with glandular fever, who should also be advised to refrain from alcohol for two months while the liver recovers from the acute injury. They should also be advised to avoid contact sport as EBV-induced hepatosplenomegaly can put them at risk of internal bleeding from any abdominal injury. If patients meet the criteria for tonsillectomy (see *tonsillectomy* section) this can be considered after the inflammation has settled – an 'interval' tonsillectomy.

PERITONSILLAR ABSCESS

Also known as a quinsy, a peritonsillar abscess is a collection of pus that develops between the tonsillar capsule and the surrounding superior constrictor muscle. This condition mainly occurs in young adults, either spontaneously or as a result of acute tonsillitis.

On examination, the patient has trismus (an inability to fully open the mouth), and the uvula is pushed away from the midline by the swelling under the soft palate. If large, a quinsy may cause airway compromise.

The soft palate is first sprayed with local anaesthetic, and the collection aspirated to confirm the presence of pus. A 19G white needle on a luer-lock and 10 or 20 mL syringe is used (1 cm of the tip of the needle sheath can be cut off and the remainder of the sheath replaced on the needle to act as a guard preventing over-insertion). The needle is pointed towards the back of the mouth (rather than drifting laterally), and the area of maximal fluctuance aspirated (or on an arc between a third of the way, and half way from the base of the uvula to the last upper molar).

Incision and drainage can be performed in the same location using a no.11 blade with tape wrapped around the blade to expose only the distal 1 cm. The incision can be opened by the use of Tilley's dressing forceps, and a Yankauer sucker can be used to remove the purulent material.

Patients are usually admitted and treated as for severe tonsillitis with intravenous antibiotics, although where symptoms completely resolve after drainage, outpatient antibiotic therapy may be sufficient. It is helpful to send a sample to microbiology to guide antibiotic therapy although patients are usually managed with benzylpenicillin and metronidazole.

SUPRAGLOTTITIS

Supraglottitis is inflammation of the soft tissues immediately above the vocal cords. It is normally caused by *Haemophilus influenzae, Streptococcus pneumoniae* or *Streptococcus pyogenes.* Patients usually complain of a short history of a sore throat with rapid hoarseness and dysphagia. This may be sufficiently severe to prevent them from swallowing their saliva.

These patients must be assessed as a priority as the airway can rapidly deteriorate. Shortness of breath, tachypnoea or stridor are worrying features and a senior ENT and anaesthetic input should always be sought. Flexible nasolaryngoscopy should be performed with caution where significant airway obstruction is present. Depending on the severity of the airway compromise patients may be nursed in ITU or a high dependency unit but the milder cases may be observed in an easily-visible 'airway' bed on an ENT ward.

Adrenaline nebulisers (1 mL of 1:1000, or diluted in 4 mL of normal saline) are effective in reducing some of the mucosal swelling. Heliox (Helium/oxygen) provides relief as this low density gas increases flow. Patients should be cannulated and given intravenous dexamethasone 8 mg or hydrocortisone 200 mg to help reduce mucosal oedema, although this only works fully after a few hours. Intravenous 3rd generation cephalosporins are normally the antibiotic of choice. These patients may need intervention to secure their airway such as intubation, tracheostomy under local anaesthesia, or emergency cricothyroidotomy.

EPIGLOTTITIS

Severe inflammation of the epiglottis in children is fortunately now rare as a result of the *Haemophylus influenzae* Type B vaccine (20, 21).

Children present with stridor; drooling is common, and 'sitting upright' (in the 'sniffing the morning air' position) to maximize the available airway.

Any potential stimulant can send them into complete airway obstruction. These children should <u>not</u> be examined nor cannulated. A Senior anaesthetist and ENT surgeon must be called. The patient is taken to theatre in order to secure the airway by intubation, although an emergency tracheostomy may occasionally be required. Patients are kept intubated and treated with intravenous antibiotics until a leak around the cuff of the endotracheal tube is observed, an indication of decreased airway swelling.

SMOKE INHALATION

Patients who have been exposed to dense smoke are often admitted under chest physicians. The upper airway must not be neglected. The effects of smoke injury on the larynx can develop over several hours and these patients should be closely monitored in hospital in a high dependency setting. Singeing of the nasal hair and soot on the nasal or oral mucosa and voice change indicate smoke inhalation. Nasolaryngoscopy should be performed to visualize the larynx and this may need to be repeated if symptoms deteriorate. Steroids can be useful in reducing mucosal oedema. These patients should be discussed with a senior promptly, because development of marked laryngeal inflammation may prevent intubation and necessitate a tracheostomy to secure the airway.

PARAPHARYNGEAL ABSCESS

An abscess may form within the parapharyngeal space. This is an inverted pyramidal space bounded superiorly by the skull base, medially the pharynx, posteriorly by the prevertebral muscles, laterally by the mandible and parotid fascia, with its apex at the greater cornu of the hyoid bone.

Infection may arise from a dental or pharyngeal source (commonly tonsil). The carotid sheath runs through the parapharyngeal space and therefore, infections in this area can lead to thrombosis of the great vessels or airway compromise (22). Patients report throat discomfort, unilateral neck swelling with limitation of movement, and may have trismus. There will be a palpable swelling in the upper neck near the angle of the jaw, with medialisation of the oropharynx. History and examination findings should help to identify the initial source of the infection and antibiotics (normally a cephalosporin and metronidazole) should be commenced intravenously. Patients require a contrast enhanced CT scan to confirm the presence of a collection and to plan potential surgical drainage (these include an external neck approach, or via a transoral route following excision of the tonsil). Patients should, therefore, remain starved until discussed with a senior colleague.

RETROPHARYNGEAL ABSCESS

In the absence of a penetrating foreign body, a retropharyngeal abscess normally occurs in children and results from necrotic degeneration of a retropharyngeal lymph node. In adults they can rarely result from the spread of spinal tuberculosis (22). Patients present with stridor, neck stiffness, pain, and dysphagia. Protrusion of the posterior pharyngeal wall can be seen on nasendoscopic examination. A full blood count with inflammatory markers and a lateral soft tissue neck radiograph will help confirm the diagnosis, but a CT scan of the neck with contrast is required.

In some situations, a tracheostomy is first performed under local anaesthetic in order to secure the airway, before the abscess is drained via a per-oral route.

FOREIGN BODIES (UPPER AERO-DIGESTIVE TRACT)

Oral cavity – Foreign bodies are usually easily visible on examination with a headlight. It is also possible to palpate the floor of the mouth, tongue and other structures to identify a foreign body. The foreign body can be carefully removed per-orally with conventional instruments.

Oropharynx – Foreign bodies, typically fish bones, may not be readily visible. Careful examination of the tonsils, posterior pharyngeal wall, tongue base and valleculae is essential, using both the headlight and flexible nasoendoscope. Visual examination is typically sufficient to exclude a foreign body. However, a lateral soft tissue x-ray is indicated, although some fish bones are not radio-opaque (23). Foreign bodies can be carefully removed per-orally using Magill forceps.

Hypopharynx/oesophagus – Foreign bodies ranging from meat or fish bones, soft food bolus to batteries and coins can obstruct in this region. Patients will complain of a foreign body sensation, pain, dysphagia or drooling. If the foreign body is above the cricopharyngeus, patients can reliably locate the site of impaction (24).

The most common sites of oesophageal obstruction are at the:

- Cricopharyngeus.
- Arch of aorta.
- Tracheal bifurcation.
- Gastro-oesophageal junction.

The hypopharynx can be examined with the flexible nasoendoscope looking carefully in the pyrifom fossae and post-cricoid region. Pooling of saliva in the hypopharynx is suggestive of an oesophageal foreign body.

If the foreign body is not easily visualized in the hypopharynx or oesophagus a soft tissue neck film or chest film (anterior posterior (AP) and lateral) is required. Where a fish bone is difficult to locate CT is more accurate (25, 26).

If the bolus contains no bony or sharp material, these can be initially managed with fizzy drinks or pineapple juice. Buscopan or diazepam can relieve any spasm and allow the bolus to pass into the stomach. If a soft bolus is in the lower oesophagus, then a flexible oesophagogastroduodenoscopy (OGD) is a safer option to push the bolus into the stomach.

If the foreign body is a bone, sharp fragment or non-organic, especially a battery, then removal is required urgently to avoid oesophageal

perforation and subsequent complications, including parapharyngeal or mediastinal abscess, which can be fatal.

Larynx/Trachea – A foreign body in the larynx or trachea can cause stridor, voice change, choking, cyanosis, difficulty breathing, tachypnoea and pneumonia. In an emergency, where total or partial obstruction causes compromise, a back slap or abdominal thrust (Heimlich manoeuvre) is employed (27).

In stable patients suspected of having inhaled a foreign body, further investigation is mandatory. In young children, the distinction between ingestion and inhalation is often blurred and they should undergo both chest PA inspiration and expiration views and abdominal films. A senior opinion is sought regarding the need for formal endoscopy, which is highly likely.

Most inhaled foreign bodies enter the trachea and then lodge in the right main bronchus.

Foreign bodies at the laryngeal inlet can be removed using an anaesthetic laryngoscope and Magill forceps. Foreign bodies in the trachea and main bronchus require formal tracheo-bronchoscopy.

LEAKAGE OR LOSS OF TRACHEOESOPHAGEAL VOICE PROSTHESIS

The speech and language therapist or ENT specialist nurse usually undertakes the routine management of the voice prosthesis in patients who have undergone laryngectomy. It is important, however, that all ENT doctors are able to manage a leaking voice prosthesis or inadvertent dislodgement.

In all cases of leakage the patient should be advised to remain nil by mouth until after appropriate assessment to minimize aspiration. To assess the leakage ask the patient to swallow a small sip of coloured fluid (e.g., coloured cordial or food dye

in water) while carefully looking at the valve and stoma with a headlight.

Central leakage through the voice prosthesis is the most common. This signifies damage to the valve by *Candida* colonization or inadvertent damage during cleaning of the voice prosthesis. The problem is resolved by fitting a new voice prosthesis by an appropriately trained healthcare professional. If no one is available, the patient is kept nil by mouth and a fine bore feeding tube can be passed through the lumen of the voice prosthesis or a nasogastric tube placed for feeding until a new voice prosthesis can be fitted. If this becomes a recurrent problem, then consideration can be given to fitting a more expensive, anti-fungal voice prosthesis (28, 29).

Peripheral leakage around the voice prosthesis is less common and potentially more difficult to resolve. Leakage is caused by the tracheoesophageal puncture (TEP) becoming larger than the voice prosthesis. This can be related to tumour recurrence or infection, which must be excluded. A number of techniques are available to the appropriately trained individual, including fitting a larger voice prosthesis, allowing the TEP to shrink and using a smaller voice prosthesis or even removing the voice prosthesis and allowing the TEP to close. If no one suitable is available, the patient is kept nil by mouth and a fine bore feeding tube can be passed through the lumen of the voice prosthesis or a nasogastric tube placed for feeding until they can be appropriately managed.

If a patient inadvertently dislodges the voice prosthesis, most are taught to pass a dilator, 14Fr Jacques or Foley catheter to keep the TEP patent or to attend hospital for the same. If the voice prosthesis is not located, then it is prudent to pass a nasoendoscope via the stoma to ensure that the voice prosthesis has not been inhaled. A new voice prosthesis can be fitted by an appropriately trained healthcare professional.

REFERENCES

1 McCarter DF, Courtney AU, Pollart SM (2007). Cerumen impaction. *Am Fam Physician* 2007; **75**:1523–8.

2 Burton MJ, Doree C (2009). Ear drops for the removal of ear wax. Cochrane Database of Systematic Reviews 1: CD004326.

3 SIGN. Diagnosis and management of childhood otitis media in primary care. Available at: www .sign.ac.uk/guidelines/fulltext/66/index. html.

4 NICE. Surgical management of children with otitis media with effusion (OME). Available at: guidance.nice.org.uk/CG60.

5 Geva A, Oestreicher-Kedem Y, Fishman G, Landsberg R, DeRowe A (2008). Conservative management of acute mastoiditis in children. *Int J Pediatr Otorhinolaryngol* **72**: 629–34.

6 Jones SEM, Mahendran S (2004). Interventions for acute auricular haematoma. Systematic Reviews 2: CD004166.

7 Davidi E, Paz A, Duchman H, Luntz M, Potasman I (2011). Perichondritis of the auricle: analysis of 114 cases. *Isr Med Assoc J* **13**: 21–4.

8 O'Malley MR, Haynes DS (2008). Sudden Hearing Loss. *Otolaryngol Clin N Am* **41**: 633–49.

9 Wei BPC, Mubiru S, O'Leary S (2006). Steroids for idiopathic sudden sensorineural hearing loss. Cochrane Database of Systematic Reviews 1: CD003998. DOI: 10.1002/14651858. CD003998.pub2.

10 Agarwal L, Pothier DD (2009). Vasodilators and vasoactive substances for idiopathic sudden sensorineural hearing loss. Cochrane Database of Systematic Reviews 4: CD003422. DOI: 10.1002/14651858.CD003422.pub4.

11 Bennett MH, Kertesz T, Perleth M, Yeung P (2007). Hyperbaric oxygen for idiopathic sudden sensorineural hearing loss and tinnitus. Cochrane Database of Systematic Reviews 1: CD004739. DOI: 10.1002/14651858.CD004739. pub3.

12 Danner CJ (2008). Facial Nerve Paralysis. *Otolaryngol Clin N Am* **41**: 619–32.

13 Sullivan FM, Swan IR, Donnan PT *et al* (2009). A randomised controlled trial of the use of aciclovir and/or prednisolone for the early treatment of Bell's palsy: the BELLS study. *Health Technol Assess* **13**(47): iii–iv, ix–xi 1–130.

14 Uscategui T, Doree C, Chamberlain IJ, Burton MJ (2008). Antiviral therapy for Ramsay Hunt syndrome (herpes zoster oticus with facial palsy) in adults. Cochrane Database of Systematic Reviews 4: CD006851. DOI: 10.1002/14651858. CD006851.pub2.

15 Uscategui T, Doree C, Chamberlain IJ, Burton MJ (2008). Corticosteroids as adjuvant to antiviral treatment in Ramsay Hunt syndrome (herpes zoster oticus with facial palsy) in adults. Cochrane Database of Systematic Reviews 3: CD006852. DOI: 10.1002/14651858. CD006852.pub2.

16 Little SC, Kesser BW (2006). Radiographic classification of temporal bone fractures: clinical predictability using a new system. *Arch Otolaryngol Head Neck Surg* **132**: 1300–4.

17 Purohit N, Ray S, Wilson T, Chawla OP (2008). The 'parent's kiss': an effective way to remove paediatric nasal foreign bodies. *Ann R Coll Surg Engl* **90**: 420–22.

18 Chadha NK, Repanos C, Carswell AJ (2009). Local anaesthesia for manipulation of nasal fractures: systematic review. *J Laryngol Otol* **123**: 830–6.

19 Ketcham AS, Han JK (2010). Complications and management of septoplasty. *Otolaryngol Clin North Am* **43**: 897–904.

20 Guardiani E, Bliss M, Harley E (2010). Supraglottitis in the era following widespread immunisation against Haemophilus influenzae type B: evolving principle in diagnosis and management. *Laryngoscope* **120**: 2183–8.

21 Sobol SE, Zapata S (2008). Epiglottitis and Croup. *Otolaryngol Clin N Am* **41**: 551–66.

22 Vieira F, Allen SM, Stocks RM, Thompson JW (2008). Deep neck infection. *Otolaryngol Clin N Am* **41**: 459–83.

23 Ell SR, Parker AJ (1992). The radio-opacity of fishbones. *Clinical Otolaryngology and Allied Sciences* **17**(6): 514–16.

24 Connolly AAP, Birchall M, Walsh-Waring GP, Moore-Gillon V (1992). Ingested foreign bodies: patient-guided localization is a useful clinical tool. *Clinical Otolaryngology and Allied Sciences* **17**(6): 520–24.

25 Lue AJ, Fang WD, Manolidis S (2000) Use of plain radiography and computed tomography to identify fish bone foreign bodies. *Otolaryngology Head and Neck Surgery* **123**(4): 435–38.

26 Shrime MG, Johnson PE, Stewart MG (2007). Cost-effective diagnosis of ingested foreign bodies. *The Laryngoscope* **117**(5): 785–93.

27 UK Resuscitation Council (2010). Adult Basic Life Support. Resuscitation Guidelines: 25–6.

28 Leder SB, Acton LM, Kmiecik J, *et al* (2005). Voice restoration with the advantage tracheoesophageal voice prosthesis. Otolaryngol Head Neck Surg **133**(5): 681–84.

29 Soolsma J, van den Brekel MW, Ackerstaff AH, *et al* (2008). Long-term results of Provox ActiValve, solving the problem of frequent candida- and 'underpressure'- related voice prosthesis replacements. *Laryngoscope* **118**(2): 252–57.

4

EPISTAXIS

This common ENT emergency has been estimated to affect 7–14% of the population, although ENT specialists see only approximately 6% of all cases (1). Patients may present in the acute setting or be seen on an elective basis in the outpatient clinic with recurrent episodes of epistaxis.

ANATOMY

Multiple branches of both the internal and external carotid arteries supply the nose, through multiple anastamoses. The internal carotid artery, via the ophthalmic artery, supplies the roof of the nasal cavity by the anterior and posterior ethmoidal arteries. The external carotid artery supplies the nasal cavity via the sphenopalatine, greater palatine and superior labial arteries (2).

Most epistaxes arise from septal vessels rather than those of the lateral wall of the nose. The most common area to bleed is Little's area the anterior septum, also known as Kiesselbach's plexus (Figure 4.1) (3).

Although Woodruff's plexus has been described as a common site of posterior bleeding (4) (a venous plexus located inferior to the posterior end of the inferior turbinate), it is now accepted that even posterior bleeds are more likely to be septal than from the lateral nasal wall (5).

AETIOLOGY

Epistaxis can be classified into primary (idiopathic) or secondary (6). Around 80% of epistaxes are idiopathic. Causative factors can be divided into local and systemic (Table 4.1).

The most commonly identified local cause of epistaxis is trauma – digital, surgical or accidental. Other local causes include infection, inflammation, foreign body, endocrine (e.g., during pregnancy), benign (e.g., juvenile nasopharyngeal angiofibroma) or malignant (sinonasal tumours), neoplastic or environmental (e.g., airborne particulate matter) (7).

Systemic causes include: hypertension, antiplatelet or anticoagulant drugs (e.g., aspirin, clopidogrel, warfarin, heparin), haematological disorders such as haemophilia, leukaemia, thrombocytopenia and hereditary haemorrhagic telangectasia (HHT).

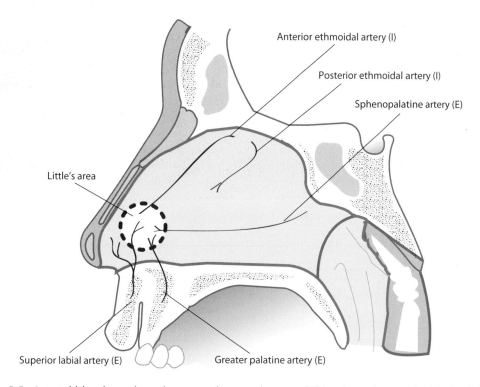

Figure 4.1. Arterial blood supply to the nose. The nose has a rich blood supply, supplied by both internal (I) and external (E) carotid arteries. Little's area, or Kiesselbach's plexus, represents a confluence of these vessels.

Table 4.1. Local and systemic causes of epistaxis.

Local	Systemic Disorders
Trauma	Hypertension
Infection (e.g., upper respiratory tract infection (URTI), acute sinusitis)	Drugs (e.g., aspirin, warfarin)
Foreign body	Haematological disorders: Myelomas Leukaemia Haemophilia Hepatic disorders
Chemical irritants	Genetic conditions (e.g., hereditary haemorrhagic telangectasia (HHT)
Neoplastic disorders Benign/malignant neoplasm Juvenile angiofibroma	

HISTORY

In the elective outpatient setting this can be taken at leisure; in an acute bleed it is often taken while treatment is being initiated. Important points about the bleeding itself include onset, duration, side (may often start on one side then appear to become bilateral due to overflow), whether anterior (running out of the nose) or posterior (swallowing blood), or both, with profuse bleeding; previous episodes and any treatment given; precipitating factors including recent trauma or surgery. If trauma is involved, significant head injury must be excluded. In the past medical history, key factors include hypertension, coagulopathies and HHT. Relevant drugs include antihypertensives, aspirin, warfarin and heparin. Social history is important as it may determine whether a patient is safe to be discharged after a potentially heavy bleed. Frail elderly patients living alone may not be.

MANAGEMENT

Never underestimate this ENT emergency. Always begin with the Airway, Breathing, Circulation (ABC) algorithm:

Airway – If compromised, assess the oropharynx and suction any clots.
Breathing
Circulation – Ensure wide-bore intravenous access and send blood for a full blood count and group and save (G&S) in all but minor cases; routine coagulation screens are not indicated in the absence of relevant risk factors (8). Check heart rate and blood pressure and resuscitate with fluids and/or blood as required. Remember that young patients may maintain a normal pulse rate and blood pressure until in severe shock. Estimate blood loss and instigate simple first aid measures with firm compression of both nostrils, head tilted forward, and apply ice to the back of the patient's neck.

EXAMINATION

In the outpatient clinic, or if the acute bleed has settled, this can be done thoroughly. In the acute situation it may not be possible to examine the patient fully, depending on the degree of bleeding.

If you are able to do so, begin with anterior rhinoscopy using a Thudichum's speculum and headlight. This allows inspection of the anterior septum and in particular Little's area, a likely site of the bleeding vessel. If no obvious bleeding point is seen and the situation permits, complete the examination using a rigid Hopkins rod endoscope to evaluate the nasal cavities and postnasal space.

In emergency situations, wear gloves, an eye shield and an apron or gown. Suction is usually required during examination and treatment. Other equipment needs to be available to allow further management as detailed below.

TREATMENT

It is important to correct hypertension and over-anticoagulation. Medical or haematological input may be required in difficult cases. Thrombocytopenia is corrected with platelet transfusion and packs avoided in these cases if possible as they cause further trauma to the nasal mucosa with inevitable re-bleeding on pack removal. Absorbable packs, such as oxidized cellulose or gelatine sponge soaked in adrenaline or tranexamic acid, are a useful alternative. There is little to be gained from stopping aspirin therapy as the half-life of platelets is seven days, but if a warfarinized patient has an elevated international normalized ratio (INR), then withholding warfarin is advisable until the bleeding is controlled and the INR back in the therapeutic range. The use of low-dose diazepam has been advocated in the past, particularly in anxious hypertensive patients, but there is little evidence for its use and controlling the epistaxis is more effective in reducing both blood pressure and anxiety (9).

CAUTERY

Cautery aims to identify and seal the bleeding vessel. This allows control of the epistaxis, avoids packing and in many cases allows the patient to be discharged after a period of observation. As most bleeding vessels arise in Little's area, cautery is often possible with anterior rhinoscopy and a silver nitrate cautery stick.

After identifying the bleeding vessel, apply topical anaesthesia, ideally combined with a vasoconstrictor to keep the field as dry as possible (e.g., co-phenylcaine – 5% lidocaine with 0.5% phenylephrine). This can be applied directly to the vessel on cotton wool. Silver nitrate cautery of the vessel is then performed directly; if it is an 'end-on' vessel, it can be helpful to cauterize around it before touching the vessel itself. Naseptin cream (0.1%

chlorhexidine dihydrochloride, 0.5% neomycin sulphate) is applied to the cauterized area twice daily for 1–2 weeks. An alternative, such as chloramphenicol ointment, should be used in patients with peanut allergy, as Naseptin contains arachis (peanut) oil.

If an obvious vessel or bleeding point is not seen anteriorly, it may be possible to examine more posteriorly with a rigid endoscope, again after topical anaesthesia/vasoconstriction. While the use of silver nitrate cautery is possible for posterior epistaxis, it is more difficult to be precise and avoid touching other parts of the nose with the stick (10). If available, bipolar electrocautery is more practical for use with an endoscope, allowing diathermy of the specific bleeding point (11).

ANTERIOR NASAL PACKING

If the epistaxis is not controlled with simple measures, then packing is required. In the first instance this is anterior nasal packing, which is most commonly performed with a nasal tampon (Figure 4.2). Various packs are available, from simple sponges such as Merocel™ to newer, self-lubricating, hydrocolloid-covered packs such as Rapid Rhino™.

The insertion technique is the same for all nasal packs. Elevate the nasal tip with one hand and firmly push the pack in along the floor of the nose with the other. It is preferable to support the back of the patient's head to facilitate complete insertion in one smooth movement. Ensure that the pack is inserted parallel to the palate as the nasal cavity runs straight back, not upwards. Once in place, sponges need to be expanded with a little water; newer devices may have a concealed balloon that requires inflation.

Unilateral packing of the bleeding side may be sufficient. However, the expanded pack may push the septum across without providing adequate compression. If bleeding does continue, insert a contralateral pack.

Anterior packing may also be performed with a long length of ribbon gauze soaked in bismuth iodoform paraffin paste (BIPP). This is layered into the nose, along its whole length, using Tilley dressing forceps (Figure 4.3). This is not a pleasant experience for the patient, whose head will need

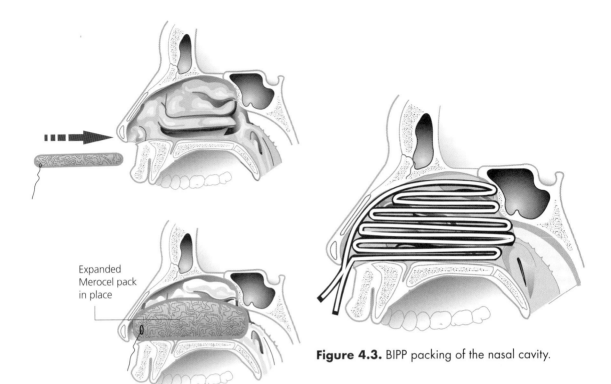

Figure 4.3. BIPP packing of the nasal cavity.

Expanded
Merocel pack
in place

Figure 4.2. Insertion of a Merocel nasal tampon.

to be supported during the packing, but it can be a very effective way of providing more compression than nasal tampons.

It is standard practice in most departments to admit patients once they have been packed for observation and pack removal after 24 hours if stable. However, local protocols will be in place and some patients may be discharged with their pack(s) *in situ*, to return for follow-up and pack removal in the outpatient department (12).

POSTERIOR NASAL PACKING

If bleeding continues despite adequate anterior nasal packing, the next step is a posterior pack. There are various commercial balloon devices designed for this (Figure 4.4). Although not licensed, in some situations a female Foley catheter can be used (size 12 or 14 French). The catheter is passed along the the floor of the nose until the tip is seen behind the soft palate. Once inflated with 5–10 mL of water (not saline as this can corrode the balloon), the catheter is gently pulled into the posterior choana. The catheter is clipped to prevent deflation of the balloon and to hold it in place; an umbilical clip or a simple artery clip can be used. An anterior BIPP pack is placed round the catheter. It is essential to ensure that the catheter or umbilical clip does not rest on the

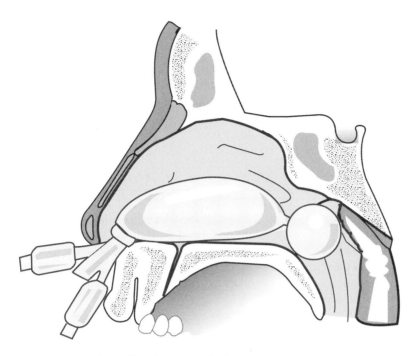

Figure 4.4. Position of an inflated epistaxis balloon.

nares as they can rapidly cause pressure necrosis of the alar rim with subsequent notching. Gauze or cotton wool can be used to protect the alar margin.

Other complications reported with posterior nasal packing have been respiratory (such as obstructive sleep apnoea), vagal (from nasopharyngeal stimulation) and cardiac (including myocardial infarction) (13).

Packs, either anterior or posterior, are left in for 24 hours and no longer than 48 hours. If the patient has any risk factors for endocarditis or has required repacking, oral antibiotic cover (e.g., amoxicillin) is given while packs are in place.

SURGICAL INTERVENTION

EUA

If bleeding remains uncontrolled, or if the patient bleeds again after removal of their pack, an examination under anaesthetic is required with a view to cautery or vessel ligation as indicated, or rarely more formal posterior nasal packing.

Septoplasty may be required if there is significant deviation or a large septal spur; this may have prevented adequate packing initially. If an obvious bleeding point is seen, it can be cauterized with bipolar diathermy.

VESSEL LIGATION

Endoscopic sphenopalatine artery (SPA) ligation is now commonly employed as the primary surgical procedure for epistaxis when operative intervention is required (14). The SPA is the major blood supply to the posterior aspect of the nasal cavity and may have multiple branches that require ligating individually.

Transantral maxillary artery ligation, via a Caldwell Luc approach, has become less popular with the advent of the endoscopic SPA technique, which is much less invasive.

If SPA or maxillary artery ligation fails to control bleeding, or in cases of traumatic epistaxis (with possible ethmoid fracture), the anterior and posterior ethmoid arteries can be ligated. This is performed via an external approach using a modified Lynch-Howarth incision.

If bleeding continues despite these measures, then the external carotid artery may be ligated in the neck (15).

EMBOLIZATION

Some centres will have access to radiological embolization. This may be employed if other measures have failed or if general anaesthesia has to be avoided due to significant comorbidities. Patients must be actively bleeding for this procedure to be effective, as angiography is required to identify the bleeding vessel before particulate embolization can be performed. Patients are warned of the risk of stroke and skin and palate necrosis (16).

See Figure 4.5 for a basic treatment algorithm for epistaxis.

HEREDITARY HAEMORRHAGIC TELANGECTASIA

This autosomal dominant condition warrants specific mention, as its most common symptom is nosebleeds. Patients are well educated and will often not seek medical treatment unless the bleeding becomes severe or protracted. Cautery, standard packing and surgical ligation of vessels should be avoided if at all possible. If packing is required, an absorbable pack such as a gelatine sponge soaked in adrenaline is the most appropriate method, as the nasal mucosa in these patients is very fragile and will be further traumatized by pack insertion and subsequent removal. If formal packing is required, it should ideally be removed in theatre under general anaesthetic, when KTP or an argon laser can be used to target the individual lesions, or more definitive treatment such as septodermoplasty or even nasal closure can be performed (17). Vessel ligation and embolization tend to provide only a temporary solution, but may allow time to arrange more specific treatment as above. Such cases may require discussion with a specialist centre.

> ### KEY POINTS:
>
> 1 Epistaxis is a common problem that is potentially life-threatening; resuscitation may be required.
> 2 Visualization and cautery of the bleeding point are often successful, as most primary epistaxis arises from the anterior septum.
> 3 Anterior and/or posterior nasal packing may be required to control profuse bleeding.
> 4 Recalcitrant cases will require timely operative intervention.

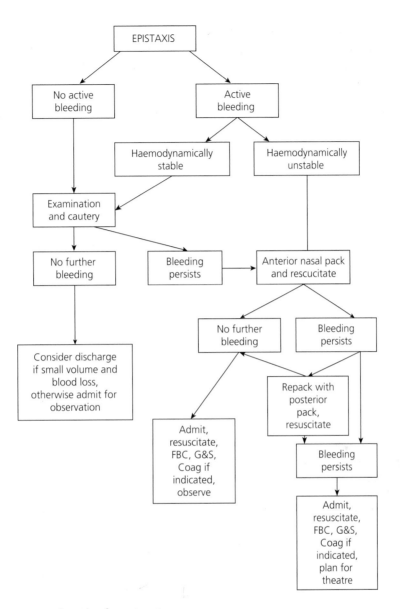

Figure 4.5. A treatment algorithm for epistaxis.

REFERENCES

1 McGarry GW (7th edition 2008). Epistaxis. In: Scott-Brown's Otorhinolaryngology Head and Neck Surgery Volume 2 Part 13. Hodder Arnold, London.

2 Janfaza P, Montgomery WM, Salman SD (2001). In: Surgical Anatomy of the Head and Neck (pp. 283–4). Lippincott Williams & Wilkins, Philadelphia.

3 Mackenzie D (1914). Little's area or the Locus Kiesselbachi. *Journal of Laryngology* 1: 21–2.

4 Woodruff GH (1949). Cardiovascular epistaxis and the naso-nasopharyngeal plexus. *Laryngoscope* **15**: 1238–47.

5 Chiu TW, Shaw-Dunn J, McGarry GW (1998). Woodruff's nasopharyngeal plexus: how important is it in posterior epistaxis? *Clinical Otolaryngology* **23**: 272–9.

6 Melia L, McGarry GW (2011). Epistaxis: update on management. *Current Opinion in Otolaryngology Head and Neck Surgery* **19**: 30–5.

7 Bray D, Monnery P, Toma AG (2004). Airborne environmental pollutant concentration and hospital epistaxis presentation: a 5-year review. *Clinical Otolaryngology* **29**: 655–8.

8 Shakeel M, Trinidade A, Iddamalgoda T, *et al* (2010). Routine clotting screen has no role in the management of epistaxis: reiterating the point. *European Archives of Otorhinolaryngology* **267**: 1641–4.

9 Thong JF, Lo S, Houghton R, Moore-Gillon V (2007). A prospective comparative study to examine the effects of oral diazepam on blood pressure and anxiety levels in patients with acute epistaxis. *Journal of Laryngology and Otology* **121**: 124–9.

10 Webb CJ, Beer H (2004). Posterior nasal cautery with silver nitrate. *Journal of Laryngology and Otology* **118**: 713–14.

11 Ahmed A, Woolford TJ (2003). Endoscopic bipolar diathermy in the management of epistaxis: an effective and cost-efficient treatment. *Clinical Otolaryngology* **28**: 273–5.

12 Van Wyk FC, Massey S, Worley G, Brady S (2007). Do all epistaxis patients with a nasal pack need admission? A retrospective study of 116 patients managed in accident and emergency with a peer-reviewed protocol. *Journal of Laryngology and Otology* **121**: 222–7.

13 Rotenberg B, Tam S (2010). Respiratory complications from nasal packing: systematic review. *Journal of Otolaryngology Head and Neck Surgery* **39**: 606–14.

14 Douglas R, Wormald P (2007). Update on epistaxis. *Current Opinion in Otolaryngology Head and Neck Surgery* **15**: 180–3.

15 Srinivasan V, Sherman IW, O'Sullivan G (2000). Surgical management of intractable epistaxis: an audit of results. *Journal of Laryngology and Otology* **114**: 697–700.

16 Sadri M, Midwinter K, Ahmed A, Parker A (2006). Assessment of safety and efficacy of arterial embolization in the management of intractable epistaxis. *European Archives of Otorhinolaryngology* **263**: 560–6.

17 Lund VJ, Howard DJ (1999). A treatment algorithm for the management of epistaxis in hereditary haemorrhagic telangectasia. *American Journal of Rhinology* **13**: 319–22.

5

AUDIOLOGY

The principal function of audiological testing is to establish hearing thresholds accurately and to determine whether there is any impairment. If impairment is detected, testing is used to establish the site, type (conductive, sensorineural or mixed) and severity of the hearing loss (Figure 5.1).

Tests of hearing are divided into behavioural and objective. When presented with sound, each aspect of the auditory pathway responds in a way that can

be measured. This response may be the test subject performing a specific task to indicate hearing a sound stimulus (behavioural response) or the measurement of a physical property of the system (objective response). Objective tests do not require the active cooperation of a subject and are not a true measure of hearing, which is a subjective sensation. They do, however, allow for certain inferences to be made regarding a subject's ability to hear.

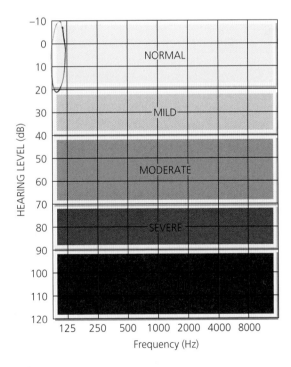

Figure 5.1. Levels of hearing loss.

BEHAVIOURAL AUDIOMETRY

∎ Pure tone audiometry

Indication

● To establish hearing thresholds

Pure tone audiometry is used to provide threshold information and to identify the presence and magnitude of any hearing loss. Thresholds are usually measured both for air conduction (via headphones) and for bone conduction (via a bone vibrator). The information provided by pure tone audiometry may be plotted graphically as an audiogram. The audiogram represents hearing sensitivity (dB HL) across a discrete frequency spectrum (125–8000 Hz). A wide variety of symbols are used to denote the findings (Figure 5.2).

O	right air conduction thresholds
X	left air conduction thresholds
Δ	unmasked bone conduction
[	right bone conduction thresholds
]	left bone conduction thresholds
↘	threshold poorer at that level, but cannot be determined because of limited output of the audiometer

Figure 5.2. Symbols commonly used in pure tone audiometry.

The reason for using a hearing level scale rather than sound pressure level (SPL) scale reflects the fact that the threshold of hearing as measured in SPL is not the same across all frequencies. For example, less energy is required to detect a 1000 Hz sound at threshold (7.5 dB SPL) than at 125 Hz (47.5 dB SPL); the resulting audiogram would be particularly difficult to interpret. The dB HL scale is a scale of human hearing where 0 dB HL reflects the threshold of hearing of an otologically normal individual irrespective of its frequency. It is against this normal hearing population that an individual's hearing is compared.

Pure tone audiometry is performed in accordance with the British Society of Audiology's recommended procedures (1). Testing is ideally carried out in a customized acoustic booth to minimize background noise. Frequency-specific sound stimuli are first delivered via headphones to test air conduction thresholds. Patients are instructed to indicate (by pressing a button) when they hear a tone, however faint. Testing begins with the better hearing ear and frequencies (250–8000 Hz) are tested in a specified order. Stimuli are initially presented at 30 dB above expected threshold. This is then increased in 20 dB steps until heard. The stimulus is then lowered in 10 dB steps until no longer heard and raised in 5 dB steps until a threshold becomes evident. There must be a minimum of two responses at that level. The threshold is marked on the audiogram with the appropriate symbol. Bone conduction thresholds are undertaken with a bone vibrator placed on the mastoid process of the ear with the worst air conduction thresholds. It is only possible to test frequencies between 250 and 4000 Hz. The maximum output of the bone vibrator is approximately 70 dB; stimulation beyond these levels may result in the vibrations being felt rather than heard.

Air conduction thresholds represent the sensitivity of the hearing mechanism as a whole (conductive, sensorineural and central components), whereas bone conduction thresholds represent the sensitivity of the hearing mechanism from the cochlear onwards. Any difference between the two thresholds is referred to as an air–bone gap (ABG). An ABG is attributed to a problem in the conduction mechanism and hence referred to as a conductive hearing loss.

In reality, sound through bone conduction reaches the cochlea in three ways:

1 Sound escapes to the external ear canal and is subsequently transferred to the cochlea through the normal middle ear mechanism.
2 Vibrations travel directly through the middle ear ossicles and then to the cochlea.
3 Vibrations reach the cochlea directly through the skull.

If there is an external or middle ear pathology resulting in a conductive hearing loss, sound will be poorly transmitted by the first two routes, resulting in poorer bone conduction thresholds than expected. This effect is greatest at 2 kHz and explains the Carhart notch seen in otosclerosis. It also explains why correcting a conductive hearing loss can result in an apparent improvement in the bone conduction thresholds.

As discussed above, pure tone audiometry presents sound to one ear at a time, and the response measured. However, in certain conditions it is not possible to be certain that the intended (test) ear is the one actually responding. In some cases the non-test ear can pick up the sound just as well or better, a phenomenon known as cross-hearing (Figure 5.3). For example, when the hearing acuity of the ears is very different it is possible that when testing the worse ear, the better ear detects the test signal more easily. In this situation special techniques (masking) are employed to 'exclude' the non-test ear.

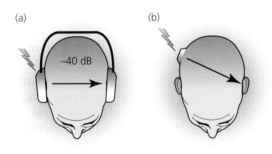

(a)   (b)

−40 dB

Figure 5.3. Transcranial attenuation through air (a) and bone conduction (b).

In order to understand cross-hearing it is necessary to understand how sound travels to the cochlea during audiological testing using the headphones and the bone vibrator. When a sound is presented via headphones to one ear, part of it escapes and vibrates the skull. This sound energy is transmitted via bone conduction to the cochlea of the opposite side and is attenuated (loses sound energy) by approximately 40 dB (Figure 5.3a).

A bone vibrator, on the other hand, will vibrate the entire skull regardless of where it is placed, with sound energy being transmitted to both cochleas with no attenuation (0 dB). It therefore corresponds to the hearing cochlea, regardless of the side tested (Figure 5.3b). For this reason, it is the sensitivity of the better hearing cochlea that determines whether masking is required, not the better hearing ear.

Three particular rules are employed to help determine whether masking is needed (2).

▮ Rules of Masking

Rule 1: When testing air conduction, if the threshold between the two ears differs by 40 dB or more at any frequency, the worse ear becomes the test ear and the better ear is masked.

Rule 2: When testing bone conduction, if the not masked bone conduction threshold at any frequency is better than the worse ear air conduction threshold by 10 dB or more, the worse ear by air conduction becomes the test ear and the better ear is masked. This provides ear-specific masked bone conduction thresholds.

Rule 3: When testing air conduction, if rule 1 has not been applied (i.e., inter-aural AC difference less than 40 dB), but the not masked bone conduction threshold is better by 40 dB, then the not masked air conduction is attributed to the worse ear. The worse ear becomes the test ear and the better ear is masked.

Interpretation of an audiogram

● Air and bone conduction thresholds equal to or better than 20 dB are considered to be within normal limits (Audiogram 5.4a). Beyond 20 dB, the degree of hearing loss is classified as mild, moderate, severe or profound (Figure 5.4a−d).

● With a pure conductive hearing loss, the ear-specific masked bone conduction threshold is normal while there is a gap of more than 10 dB between the air and bone conduction thresholds (Audiogram 5.4b). This gap is known as the air−bone gap (ABG).

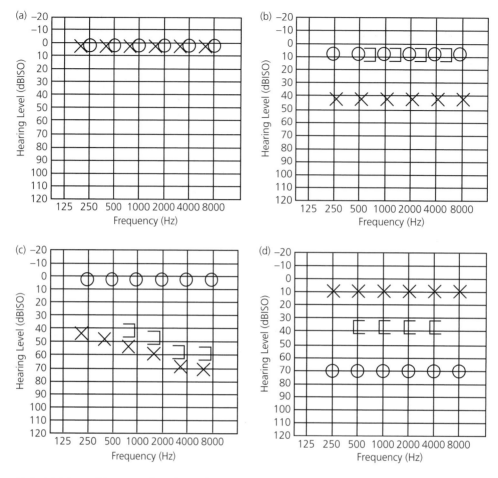

Figure 5.4. (a) Normal hearing. (b) Left conductive hearing loss. (c) Left sensorineural hearing loss. (d) Right mixed hearing loss.

- With a pure sensorineural hearing loss, both the ear-specific air and the bone conduction thresholds are worse than 20 dB, but there is no ABG (Audiogram 5.4c).
- In a mixed hearing loss, the ear-specific bone conduction thresholds are worse than 20 dB and there is an ABG greater than 10 dB (Audiogram 5.4d).
- Asymmetry in thresholds is considered significant if there is more than 10 dB difference between the ears at two adjacent frequencies.

SPEECH AUDIOMETRY

Indications:

- Functional hearing assessment (speech or word discrimination).

- To confirm conductive or sensorineural hearing loss.

- Investigation of non-organic hearing loss.

In speech audiometry, the patient is asked to repeat pre-recorded words (i.e., the Arthur Boothroyd word list) presented via a free field, headphones or bone conductor at various intensity levels. The speech audiogram graphically displays the percentage of correct responses as a function of the sound pressure level that the words were presented at (Figure 5.5). One of the variables measured is the optimum discrimination score (ODS). This is 100% in patients with normal hearing (line 1, Figure 5.5) and in patients with pure conductive hearing losses, although a conductive loss requires higher intensity levels (line 2, Figure 5.5). In sensorineural hearing losses, ODS is usually less than 100% regardless of the sound intensity (line 3, Figure 5.5). With neural losses, a phenomenon known as rollover may be observed (line 4, Figure 5.5).

Speech audiometry supplies useful information regarding a patient's hearing handicap and can guide management. An example of this is in the management of otosclerosis. When considering stapedectomy, a patient with an ODS of less than 70% must be counselled that their perceived benefit may not be as good as that of someone with a score of over 70%, even if the ABG is successfully closed. An optimum discrimination score of less than 50% is regarded as being not socially useful, which can have implications in the management of individuals with vestibular schwannoma. If optimally aided ODS in the better hearing ear is less than 50%, then an individual meets the criteria for cochlear implantation.

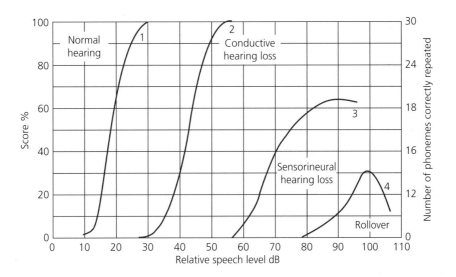

Figure 5.5. Speech audiogram.

OBJECTIVE AUDIOMETRY

▌ Tympanometry

Indications

● In conjunction with audiometry to characterize hearing loss.
● To document normal middle ear compliance.

Tympanometry is not a test of hearing but is used in conjunction with pure tone audiometry to help determine the nature of any hearing loss.

Tympanometry measures the compliance of the middle ear system. Factors influencing middle ear compliance include the integrity and mobility of the tympanic membrane and ossicular chain, the presence of fluid and middle ear pressure. Tympanometry is therefore used clinically to provide information regarding the state of the tympanic membrane, ossicular chain, middle ear cleft and Eustachian tube function.

The test involves placing a small probe in the ear canal to form an airtight seal. The probe contains a sound generator, microphone and pump, all connected to a tympanometer. A sound stimulus is passed down the ear canal to the tympanic membrane. The stimulus used is a 226 Hz probe tone unless testing infants less than four months old, for whom a 1 kHz stimulus is used. A proportion of the sound energy is transmitted through the middle ear apparatus and the rest is reflected. The probe microphone records reflected sound energy. The more compliant the middle ear system, the less energy reflected. Because the compliance of the tympanic membrane is maximal when the pressure between its two sides is equal, it is possible to measure the middle ear pressure by altering the pressure in the external ear canal via the pump channel in the ear probe.

The test generates a tympanogram. This is a graphical representation of the compliance of the tympanic membrane as a function of the change in pressure in the external ear canal. Tympanograms are most commonly described according to the Jerger system of classification (3). There are three types.

Type A – Demonstrates a well-defined peak compliance of between +100 and −150 daPa (Figure 5.6a). It signifies normal middle ear pressure.

Type B – Demonstrating no obvious peak across the pressure range (Figure 5.6b). Interpretation depends on the measured ear canal volume. This should be less than 1 cm³ in a child and less than 1.5 cm³ in an adult. If the ear canal volume is normal, the flat trace is likely to represent a middle ear effusion. If the ear canal volume is increased, then the finding is likely to represent a tympanic membrane perforation or presence of a patent grommet.

Type C – Demonstrates a well-defined compliance peak at less than −150 daPa (Figure 5.6c). This most commonly signifies Eustachian tube dysfunction or a partial middle ear effusion.

Tympanometry does not provide information about hearing and inferences must be made in conjunction with information from other tests.

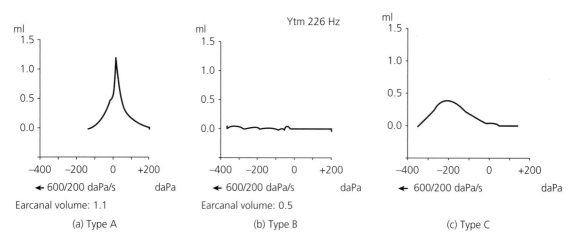

Figure 5.6. Tympanometry. (a) Normal peak. (b) No peak. (c) Negative peak.

AUDITORY EVOKED POTENTIALS

Indications

- To establish likely hearing thresholds.
- To identify cochlear or retro-cochlear pathology.

Auditory evoked potentials (AEP) describe the electrical activity within the cochlea and along the auditory pathway in response to auditory stimulation. The test involves a sound stimulus being presented to the test ear. This results in electrical activity within the auditory pathway. Scalp electrodes detect this and other non-auditory activity. The electrodes pass information to an amplifier, which amplifies and filters differences between pairs of electrodes. The stimulus is presented repeatedly and the recordings averaged. The process of amplification, filtering and averaging results in evoked potential (signal) being separated from non-auditory electrical activity (noise).

Four types of AEP are in common clinical usage:

1 Electrocochleography – This measures electrical activity within the cochlea and first-order cochlear nerve fibres in response to sound. The electrocochleogram (ECochG) records three potentials: the cochlear microphonic (CM), the summating potential (SP) and the action potential (AP). Common clinical uses include frequency-specific estimation of hearing thresholds in the very young or difficult to test and the determination of endolymphatic hydrops in Menière's disease.

2 Auditory brainstem responses (ABR) – The auditory brainstem response is a series of five waves occurring within 10 ms of a sound stimulus (Figure 5.7). Each wave is attributed to a different part of the auditory pathway from distal auditory nerve to inferior colliculus. ABR has a number of clinical uses, principally the estimation of hearing thresholds using wave V. Because the ABR is present from birth it is a useful hearing screening tool for neonates. The precise latency of each waveform has previously been exploited to detect pathology affecting the cochlear nerve, in particular as a screening test for vestibular schwannomas. In this condition there can be a delay in the latency of wave V. This has now been largely superseded by contrast-enhanced magnetic resonance imaging (MRI).

3 Auditory steady state responses (ASSR) – This is a test that uses frequency-specific stimuli modulated with respect to amplitude and frequency. Higher modulation rates generate AEP derived from the brainstem. Auditory steady state

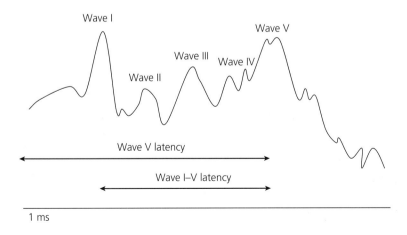

Figure 5.7. Auditory brainstem response.

responses (ASSR) analysis is based on the fact that related electrical activity coincides with the stimulus repetition rate and relies on statistical detection algorithms. The test can be used as in automated assessment of auditory thresholds.

4 Cortical auditory evoked potentials (CAEP) – Evoked potentials occurring beyond 50 ms are referred to as cortical auditory evoked potentials (CAEP). They span the transition from obligatory to cognitive responses. They can be generated using frequency stimuli. The accurate correspondence with true frequency-specific hearing thresholds make this a useful test in medico-legal assessment of hearing for compensation cases and for diagnosis in suspected non-organic hearing loss.

OTOACOUSTIC EMISSIONS

Indications

● Hearing screening.

Otoacoustic emissions (OAE) represent sound energy generated by the contraction and expansion of outer hair cells in the cochlear. These echoes can be measured by sensitive microphones placed in the ear canal. OAE are classified into two groups: spontaneous (only present in 50% of population) and evoked. Evoked OAE are emissions generated in response to a sound stimulus and are present in the majority of individuals with hearing thresholds better that 40 dB HL. In fact, OAE are present in 99% of individuals with thresholds better than 20 dB and always absent with thresholds over 40 dB. Between 20 and 40 dB there is a zone of uncertainty. For this reason they have been widely adopted as a hearing screening tool (4).

Clinically, two main types of evoked OAE are used: transient evoked OAE (TEOAE) and distortion product OAE (DPOAE). The test involves placing a small insert in the ear canal, which contains a sound generator and microphone and is attached to an OAE machine. A stimulus is generated and any ensuing emission measured. The test is performed in a quiet environment. In addition to being able to infer hearing thresholds of better than 40 dB HL, these tests provide frequency-specific information in the speech frequencies (500–4000 Hz).

Absent evoked OAE do not necessarily reflect a cochlear hearing loss and can arise if the ear canal is blocked or if there is middle ear pathology (i.e., an effusion). If OAE are genuinely absent, no inference as to the degree of loss can be made, which can range from mild (zone of uncertainty) to profound. Additionally, robust OAE may be found in individuals with auditory neuropathy spectrum disorder who may have a profound hearing loss.

KEY POINTS:

● Ensure testing equipment is maintained and meets the appropriate National Physical Laboratory calibration schedule.
● Expertise is required for both the testing and interpretation of results.
● Ensure that appropriate ear-specific information is obtained. Have masking rules been applied?
● No single test provides all the answers.
● Beware of discrepancies. Where outcomes of tests are unexpected and do not fit with observed auditory function, check that the equipment is functioning normally and that the test subject is performing the test appropriately.

✱ RECOMMENDED READING

● Browning GG (2nd edition 1998). Clinical Otology & Audiology. Butterworth-Heinemann, London.
● Graham J, Baguley D (2009). Ballantyne's Deafness. Wiley-Blackwell, Chichester.

● Katz J, Medwetsky L, Buckard RF, Hood LJ (6th edition 2010). Handbook of Clinical Audiology. Lippincott Williams & Wilkins.

REFERENCES

1 British Society of Audiology (1981). Recommended procedures for pure-tone audiometry using a manually operated instrument. *British Journal of Audiology* **15**: 213–16.

2 British Society of Audiology (1986). Recommendations procedures for masking in pure tone threshold audiometry. *British Journal of Audiology* **20**: 307–14.

3 Jerger J (1970). Clinical experience with impedance audiometry. *Arch Otolaryngol* **92**: 311–24.

4 Rea PA, Gibson WP (2003). Evidence for surviving outer hair cell function in congenitally deaf ears. *Laryngoscope* **113**: 2030–4.

6

TONSILLECTOMY

Indications

- Recurrent acute tonsillitis.
- Two or more episodes of quinsy.
- Obstructive sleep apnoea.
- Possible malignancy (e.g., unilateral tonsillar enlargement or ulceration of the tonsil surface).
- In cases of the occult primary (i.e., a metastatic deposit in a neck node), tonsillectomy may be indicated in order to exclude this as a site for the primary in conjunction with a panendoscopy.
- As part of a uvulopalatopharyngoplasty performed for the treatment of snoring.
- To access a parapharyngeal abscess.
- Rarely, to access an elongated styloid process in the management of Eagle's syndrome.

Recurrent acute tonsillitis remains the commonest indication for tonsillectomy. The frequency and severity of episodes required to list a patient for this procedure varies from unit to unit. Whilst the Scottish Intercollegiate Guidelines Network (SIGN) recommendations are helpful (suggesting patients who suffer five or more episodes of tonsillitis per annum benefit from this procedure) a decision must be made on a case-by-case basis (1, 2).

PREOPERATIVE REVIEW

The vascularity of the tonsillar tissue increases significantly during an episode of tonsillitis. Many surgeons will postpone surgery if the patient has experienced true tonsillitis in the preceding 28 days even if antibiotics have been prescribed, as intra-operative haemorrhage is increased if tonsillectomy is performed.

OPERATIVE PROCEDURE

Once anaesthetized and the airway secured with an endotracheal tube (ET), a shoulder bolster is placed under the patient and the neck extended. The patient's eyes must be taped closed. A headlight is worn by the surgeon and the patient draped.

The operation is performed from the head of the operating table. A Boyle-Davis mouth gag with an appropriately sized blade is inserted and the mouth gently opened. The tongue is positioned in the midline by sweeping the tongue base with digital manipulation. Draffin rods are used to support and lift the gag. The head must remain supported on the operating table.

Secretions are cleared from the oral cavity using suction (Figure 6.1a).

In order to remove the right tonsil, Dennis-Brown or Luc's forceps are held in the surgeon's left hand

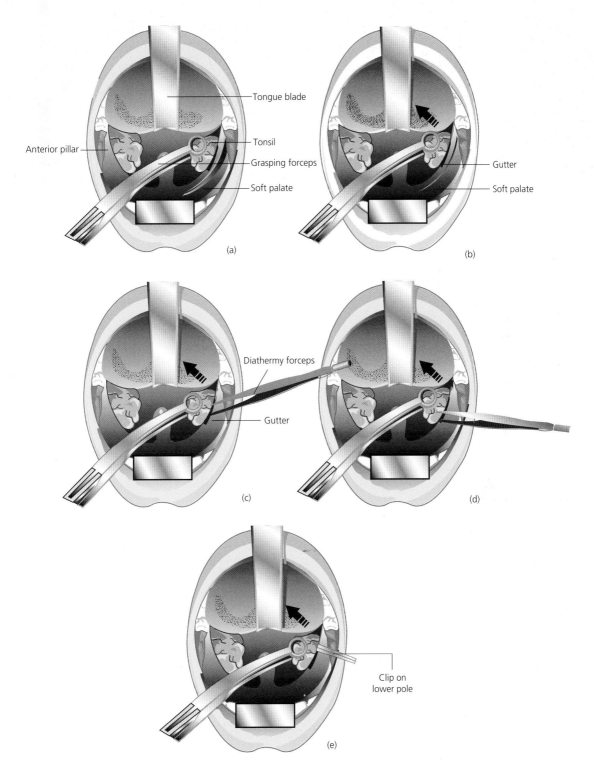

Figure 6.1. Bipolar tonsillectomy.

Labels in figure:
- Tongue blade
- Anterior pillar
- Tonsil
- Grasping forceps
- Soft palate
- (a)
- Gutter
- Soft palate
- (b)
- Diathermy forceps
- Gutter
- (c)
- (d)
- Clip on lower pole
- (e)

and the superior pole of the right tonsil is gently grasped and pulled medially (Figure 6.1b). This, in most cases, produces a visible gutter in the anterior tonsillar pillar, which marks the lateral limit of the tonsil. The mucosa is incised using McIndoe scissors or cauterized with bipolar forceps (Figure 6.3c). The scissors can then be gently inserted into the incision and opened to develop the plane between the tonsil and the superior constrictor muscle fibres. At this stage, the forceps are repositioned with the superior blade within this developed plane and the inferior blade over the medial surface of the tonsil.

A Gwyn-Evans dissector or bipolar diathermy forceps may be used to separate the muscle fibres from the white capsule of the tonsil, which should gradually peel away. Bleeding is inevitable during this part of the procedure but identifying the tonsillar capsule early and staying within the correct plane will minimize its extent. Continued traction with the forceps is the key to a clean and brisk dissection (Figure 6.1d).

As the dissection proceeds, a small 'stalk' of tissue tethers the tonsil at its inferior pole. This usually bears a significant feeding arterial vessel (the tonsillar branch of the ascending pharyngeal artery) which requires clipping with a curved Negus clip and tying with silk (Figure 6.1e). The clip is then slowly removed as the tie is thrown and the tie

then trimmed. The tonsillar fossa is packed with a tonsil swab while dissection is performed on the opposite side.

Haemostasis is achieved using bipolar diathermy or further ties. Once haemostasis has been achieved, the gag is relaxed for 30 seconds and the mouth reopened. The fossae are inspected for bleeding and dealt with accordingly. Gentle use of the sucker to remove blood from the base of the tongue and under the soft palate is accompanied by the passage of a Jacques suction catheter through the nose to remove a potential 'coroner's' clot from the postnasal space. If not removed, this clot may fall into and obstruct the airway, to be retrieved only later by the coroner. Suction is attached and the catheter gently withdrawn.

The Boyle-Davis gag is relaxed and carefully removed. The endotracheal tube may on occasion herniate into the tongue blade and hence the patient may be inadvertently extubated. This will result in a significant airway compromise and must be avoided.

A survey of the teeth must be performed to document any dental trauma (or loss which will require retrieval of the tooth). The jaw must also be assessed to exclude a temporo-mandibular joint dislocation. It is also essential to confirm that all the tonsil swabs have been removed.

POSTOPERATIVE REVIEW AND FOLLOW-UP

Patients undergoing tonsillectomy alone do not require follow-up unless tissue has been sent for histology. Whilst tonsillectomy is routinely performed as a day case procedure, those with obstructive sleep apnoea require overnight observations as an inpatient.

Patients will complain of odonophagia and otalgia, and require regular analgesia for the first postoperative week.

It is essential that patients eat and drink normally as this reduces not only the likelihood of infection but also subsequent secondary bleeding.

POST-TONSILLECTOMY HAEMORRHAGE

This is a potentially life-threatening emergency and should be managed as such. Patients must be

assessed in the Emergency Department. Assessment should include the ABC algorithm with early cannulation using wide-bore cannulae. Blood must be taken for a full blood count, clotting screen and group and save.

If the bleeding has spontaneously stopped, patients are admitted for observation.

If bleeding persists behind a tonsillar clot, this should be removed with a Yankauer sucker or Magill's forceps. A tonsil swab or ribbon gauze soaked in 1:5000 adrenaline can be held over the bleeding point and may achieve haemostasis.

If these measures fail, the patient is transferred to theatre for emergency surgical arrest of the haemorrhage. This can be achieved by diathermy or application of a tie. However, the tissue is generally friable in these situations, laying a strip of Surgicel within the tonsillar fossa and over-sewing the anterior and posterior pillars together with a heavy stitch may be required.

REFERENCES

1 Management of sore throat and indications for tonsillectomy, a national clinical guideline (April 2010). Scottish Intercollegiate Guidelines Network, Guideline 117.
2 Lowe D, Van der Meulen J, Cromwell D *et al* (2007). Key messages from the National Prospective Tonsillectomy Audit. *Laryngoscope* **117**(4): 717–24.

7

ADENOIDECTOMY

Indications

- Obstructive sleep apnoea.
- In conjunction with grommet insertion (an enlarged adenoidal pad may encroach onto the Eustachian tube orifice causing Eustachian tube dysfunction, or a biofilm may extend from the adenoidal pad onto the Eustachian tube cushion).

PREOPERATIVE REVIEW

One must always be cautious when it comes to operating on small children (<15 kg or <3 years of age) as they have a smaller circulating blood volume and a preoperative group and save sample may be required. One should exclude a personal or familial bleeding tendency and discuss this with a senior colleague if necessary. There is an increase in the vascularity of the adenoidal pad following an upper aero-digestive tract infection and many surgeons will postpone surgery if there has been a recent episode.

OPERATIVE TECHNIQUE

Two techniques are commonly used for adenoidectomy.

▌ Adenoidal curettage

Once intubated, a shoulder roll is placed under the patient to extend the neck. A headlight is required. The patient is draped, a Boyle-Davis gag inserted and the mouth opened. Once secured with Draffin rods, care should be taken to avoid damage to the teeth and lips and kinking of the endotracheal tube. A finger is inserted into the postnasal space to:

- Confirm the presence of an enlarged adenoidal pad.

- Exclude a pulsatile adenoidal pad (this may actually be an angiofibroma, in which case adenoidectomy is ill advised).
- Exclude the presence of a cleft palate or submucous cleft (an adenoidectomy may result in a nasal voice and nasal regurgitation, and is a contraindication for curette adenoidectomy).
- To exclude a choanal atresia.
- To sweep the adenoidal pad into the midline.

An adenoidal curette is passed into the postnasal space and the adenoidal pad curetted with firm but gentle pressure. The postnasal space is packed with swabs to achieve haemostasis (several swab changes may be required).

Haemostasis is confirmed by tilting the head forward and inspecting for any bleeding. Further brisk bleeding requires repacking of the postnasal space. Occasionally, suction diathermy or adrenaline-soaked packs may be required.

▐ Suction diathermy

This technique has recently gained popularity (Figure 7.1)(1, 2). Evidence suggests that suction diathermy adenoidectomy results in less intra-operative blood loss, less remnant adenoidal tissue and less postoperative nasal regurgitation of food (3).

Once anaesthetized, the patient is placed supine and a shoulder roll inserted in order to extend the neck. A Boyle-Davis mouth gag is inserted and supported with Draffin rods. Jacques catheters are passed through each nostril and the distal ends are drawn out of the oral cavity. Gentle traction is used to elevate the soft palate. A mirror is inserted into the oral cavity and used to assess the adenoidal pad. If enlarged, suction diathermy is used to cauterize the surface of the pad.

The stem of the suction diathermy is angled to allow access to the adenoidal pad. Great care is taken to avoid injury to the surrounding structures, including the Eustachian tube cushions. Adequate clearance is gained when both choanae are clearly visible and the posterior pharyngeal wall has a smooth contour. The Draffin rods are removed and the head tilted forward to allow inspection of the oropharynx for evidence of bleeding.

Complications

- Bleeding.
- Infection.
- Grisel's syndrome – atlanto-axial subluxation due to ligamentous laxity as a result of infection.

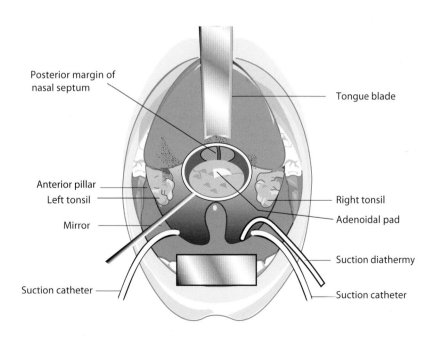

Figure 7.1. Suction diathermy of the adenoidal tissue.

POSTOPERATIVE REVIEW

Patients may develop minor neck stiffness and regular analgesia should be taken for up to a week. Prophylactic oral antibiotics may also be prescribed. If torticollis occurs, this may indicate Grisel's syndrome and the patient should return to hospital.

There is a risk of bleeding for the week following surgery, and relative isolation from other children reduces the risk of viral transmission and the development of secondary haemorrhage. In children this requires one week off school. Should bleeding occur, the patient should attend the Emergency Department immediately.

REFERENCES

1 Hartley BE, Papsin BC, Albert DM (1998). Suction diathermy adenoidectomy. *Clin Otolaryngol Allied Sci* **23**: 308–9.

2 Lo S, Rowe-Jones J (2006). How we do it: transoral suction diathermy adenoid ablation under direct vision using a 45 degree endoscope. *Clin Otolaryngol* **31**: 440–42.

3 Suction Diathermy Adenoidectomy (December 2009). NICE guidance IPG328. www.nice.org.uk/nicemedia/live/12127/46633/46633.pdf.

8

GROMMET INSERTION

Grommets are tubes placed in the tympanic membrane to ventilate the middle ear space.

Indications

- Persistent bilateral middle ear effusions resulting in >30 dB HL bilateral conductive hearing loss in two or more frequencies for at least three months.
- Recurrent acute otitis media.
- In adults, a unilateral middle ear effusion (combined with a postnasal space examination and biopsy).
- Significant tympanic membrane retraction.
- Menière's disease.

Current National Institute for Health and Clinical Excellence (NICE) guidelines (CG60 February 2008) recommend direct surgical intervention for otitis media with effusion (OME) in children up to the age of 12 years who demonstrate a hearing loss due to a persistent middle ear effusion lasting three months or more (1). However, patients must be treated on a case-by-case basis, taking into account their educational progress and speech development. Grommet insertion is not currently recommended for children with Down's syndrome, who are managed with hearing aids.

PATIENT INFORMATION AND CONSENT

The rationale for grommet insertion and alternative treatment with hearing aids should be discussed. Grommets remain in place for an average of 18 months in the paediatric age group. In 30% of children, middle ear effusions recur once the grommets have extruded.

OPERATIVE PROCEDURE

In children and most adults this procedure is performed under general anaesthetic.

The anaesthetized patient is positioned supine and the head rotated away from the operator, who is seated. A perforated ear drape is placed over the ear. The largest aural speculum that comfortably fits in the canal is used. This is held with the non-dominant hand and the microscope focused to provide a clear image of the tympanic membrane (Figure 8.1a). Any wax is removed using a Jobson-Horne probe, crocodile forceps or a Zoellner sucker. Care must be taken not to traumatize the canal mucosa. If bleeding does occur, a cotton wool pledget soaked in 1:10 000 adrenaline provides haemostasis.

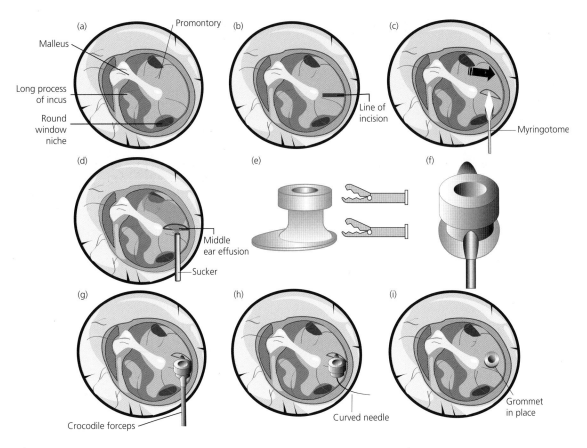

Figure 8.1. Grommet insertion.

The anteroinferior quadrant is identified and a myringotome used to make a radial incision from the umbo towards the annulus (Figure 8.1b). As the incision is performed, a note is made of the presence of an effusion and its appearance (Figure 8.1c). This is removed gently with suction using a fine end attached to a Zoellner sucker.

Forceps are used to grasp the grommet at either its rim or heel (Figure 8.1e, f). Once firmly grasped, the long axis of the grommet should be in line with the long axis of the forceps (Figure 8.1g).

The grommet is advanced such that its toe is inserted into the myringotomy incision. Gentle pressure applied at the heel of the grommet with a needle is usually required to push the grommet into place (Figure 8.1h).

A grommet inadvertently pushed into the middle ear may be retrieved by a senior colleague.

The use of topical ear drops immediately following grommet insertion has gained popularity and may reduce the incidence of grommet blockage (2).

Complications

- Recurrent ear infections, occasionally requiring removal of the grommet.
- Persistent perforation (1–2%); patients may require a myringoplasty in order to close the perforation (3).

Many surgeons advise that the ears are kept absolutely dry for at least 2 weeks after the procedure. Patients may be allowed to swim with grommets in place several weeks after insertion, unless they suffer recurrent ear infections.

Patients are reviewed after 12 weeks with repeat audiometry.

REFERENCES

1 Surgical management of children with otitis media with effusion (OME) (February 2008). NICE clinical guidance CG60. Available at: guidance.nice.org.uk/CG60.

2 Arya AK, Rea PA, Robinson PJ (2004). The use of perioperative Sofradex eardrops in preventing tympanostomy tube blockage: a prospective double-blinded randomized-controlled trial. *Clin Otolaryngol Allied Sci* **29**: 598–601.

3 Lous J, Burton MJ, Felding JU, *et al* (2005). Grommets (ventilation tubes) for hearing loss associated with otitis media with effusion in children. *Cochrane Database Syst Rev* **25**(1): CD001801.

9

SEPTOPLASTY

Nasal obstruction due to a deviated nasal septum was previously corrected by submucous resection (SMR). This involved excising much of the septal cartilage and bone at the expense of maintaining nasal support. This procedure has given way to septoplasty, which involves resection of as little septal cartilage and bone as possible (Figure 9.1), and aims to reposition it instead (1). This retains septal support and reduces the risk of postoperative septal perforation (2).

Indications

● Nasal obstruction secondary to a deviated nasal septum. Patient selection is paramount. Those with nasal obstruction due to septal deviation alone have an excellent outcome (3). If the obstruction is mainly due to mucosal disease (e.g., allergic rhinitis), then results are often less satisfactory (4).
● Cosmetic correction of a deviated nose as part of a septorhinoplasty. If there is severe deviation of the mid- and lower thirds of the nose, such as in the 'twisted nose', then an extracorporeal septoplasty technique may be required (5).
● Access for endoscopic sinonasal or skull base procedures.
● In the management of epistaxis where a deviated septum prevents adequate nasal packing.
● To obtain septal cartilage for use as an autograft.

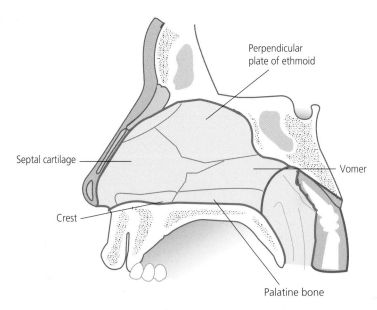

Figure 9.1. The skeleton of the nasal septum.

OPERATIVE PROCEDURE

An appropriately informed, consented and anaesthetized patient is positioned supine, head up, with a head ring for support. Topical nasal preparations such as Moffett's solution (a variable mixture of cocaine, adrenaline, normal saline and sodium bicarbonate) (6) or co-phenylcaine spray (5% lidocaine, 0.5% phenylephrine) may be instilled into the nose to improve the surgical field. The patient's eyes are taped closed or lubricating ointment instilled. The surgeon wears a headlight, although the procedure may be performed endoscopically (7).

Skin preparation is not routinely used. The patient is draped with a head towel and the whole nose exposed. The nasal cavities and septal deviation are assessed using a Killian's or Cottle's nasal speculum. It is important to identify the side and site of the deviation and relate this to the patient's obstructive symptoms (Figure 9.2).

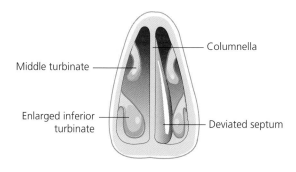

Figure 9.2. Septal deviation to the left.

A short nasal speculum is held with one blade on either side of the caudal edge of the quadrilateral cartilage, and both sides of the septum infiltrated with 2% lidocaine with 1:80 000 adrenaline using a dental syringe (Figure 9.3a–b). The mucoperichondrium should blanche following infiltration.

A no. 15 scalpel blade is used to incise the mucoperichondrium down to cartilage (Figure 9.3c–d). This incision can be placed along the caudal edge

of the quadrilateral cartilage at the septocolumellar junction (hemitransfixion incison) or approximately 0.5 cm behind the mucocutaneous junction (Killian's incision) (Figure 9.4). It is often easier to find the correct plane of dissection using a Killian's incision, but it is difficult to address caudal septal deviations through this incision. The incision is usually made on the left, but in certain cases (e.g., caudal septal dislocation to the right) the surgeon may elect to make the incision on the right.

It is important to find the correct plane for dissection; this is subperichondrial, between the cartilage and the perichondrium. It is easy to be misled and dissect the plane between perichondrium and mucosa. The perichondrium has a pale pink appearance due to its blood supply, whereas septal cartilage has a shiny white/pale blue colour. If a hemitransfixion incision has been made, sharp pointed scissors are helpful initially as the mucopericondrium is tethered anteriorly due to "McGilligan's fibres". The short nasal speculum may be pressed firmly into the incision against the cartilage to assist dissection.

A Freer's elevator is inserted between the cartilage and mucoperichondrium and the mucoperichondrial flap raised carefully along the full length of the septum (Figure 9.5). It is often easier to elevate the flap superiorly first, where it is less adherent, and continue inferiorly and posteriorly with gentle sweeping movements.

Care must be taken not to tear the flap, which can be particularly difficult over spurs or fracture lines. Another area of difficulty is at the junction of the septal cartilage and maxillary crest inferiorly, as the mucoperiosteum overlying the latter is more tightly adherent than the mucoperichondrium is to the quadrilateral cartilage, and the two are not in continuity. It is helpful to raise the mucoperiostium posteriorly over the vomer first, and then continue the dissection anteriorly with a hockey stick dissector.

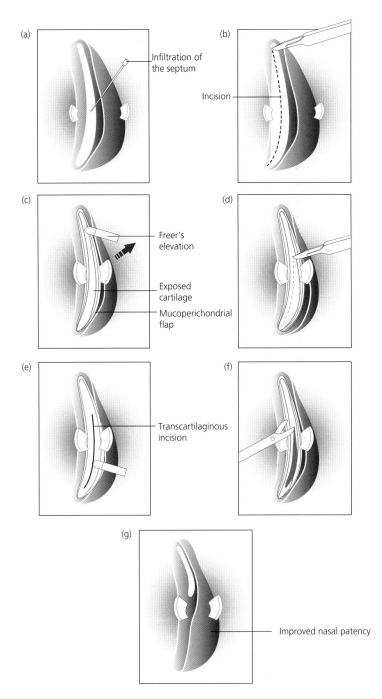

Figure 9.3. (a–g). Infiltration of the leading edge provides haemostasis (a), before an incision is made (b). A Freer's elevator is commonly used to dissect perichondrium from the septal cartilage. Once the mucoperichondrial flap has been raised, a vertical incision is made through the septal cartilage (d). A Freer's elevator is passed through the incision and the mucoperichondrium separated from the cartilage on the contralateral side (e). Turbinectomy scissors may be use to excise the cartilaginous deflection (f). The mucoperichondrial flap is separated from the cartilage and an inferior strut, shaded area, may be excised to improve nasal patency (g).

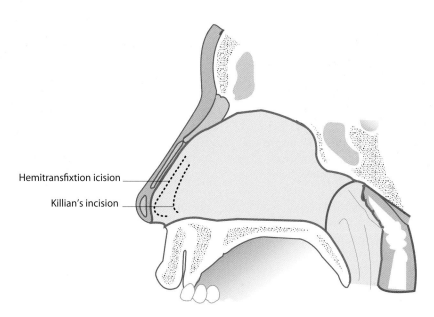

Figure 9.4. Incisions for a septoplasty. A hemitransfixtion incision is made along the anterior (leading) edge of the septum, whilst a Killian's incision is made 0.5 cm posterior to the mucocutaneous junction.

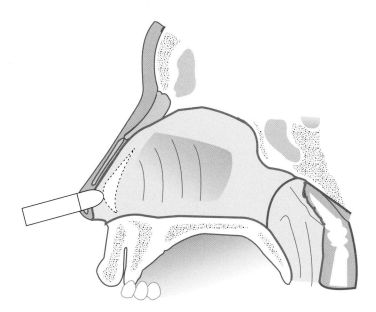

Figure 9.5. Elevation of the flap is performed with a Freer's elevator. Care must be taken to avoid a flap tear.

It is sometimes necessary to elevate a complete contralateral mucoperichondrial flap, in which case the plane can be followed over the caudal edge of the quadrilateral cartilage onto the right side and dissected as above. This is usually necessary in severe deviations only, and is avoided if possible to reduce the risk of septal perforation.

The procedure from this point will be determined by the extent of the deviation. If the quadrilateral cartilage is fixed laterally by a deviated bony septum, the osseochondral junction may be incised to release it posteriorly. The area of deviation may be amenable to resection, in which case the quadrilateral cartilage is fully incised at an appropriate point (often the most deviated part), and then a partial contralateral flap is elevated via the transcartilaginous incision (Figure 5.2e–f) to allow removal of the intervening piece of cartilage or bone. Through-cutting forceps (e.g., Jansen Middleton forceps) should be used when removing the bony septum in order to avoid twisting the perpendicular plate of the ethmoid (PPE), as there is a theoretical risk of skull base fracture at the cribriform plate and an ensuing CSF leak.

When removing quadrilateral cartilage, it is vital to understand the major areas of support that should not be resected. The most important is the keystone area; this is the junction of the quadrilateral cartilage, PPE, nasal bones and upper lateral cartilages. The cartilage and bone should not be completely separated at this point to avoid dorsal collapse. It is advisable to leave at least 1 cm dorsal and caudal struts of septal cartilage for support, although in practice one should aim to leave much more cartilage in place if feasible. Bony spurs inferiorly may be resected using a fishtail gouge. Septal cartilage may be incised or scored in order to help repositioning, and various cutting and suturing techniques have been described, particularly to address the most difficult problem of caudal deviation (8, 9).

Once the deviation has been corrected, the incision is closed with an absorbable suture. The same suture can be used to 'quilt' the septum with through-and-through mattress sutures. This reduces the risk of septal haematoma formation by closing the dead space. Nasal packing is not routinely inserted.

POSTOPERATIVE REVIEW

The patient can be discharged after observation according to the hospital's day surgery protocol. Discharge medication may include analgesia and nasal douches. Patients are advised to take 10–14 days off work, avoid nose-blowing for one week, sneeze with their mouth open if possible and avoid heavy lifting or strenuous exercise for two weeks. Patients may be followed up at three months.

Complications

- Bleeding – Some oozing is normal but heavy epistaxis requires return to hospital and may warrant nasal packing. If a septal haematoma develops, it will require draining and nasal packing.
- Infection.
- Ongoing symptoms – Either related to persistent or recurrent deviation as septal cartilage has 'memory', or to concurrent mucosal disease.
- Septal perforation – Usually asymptomatic, but may cause crusting, bleeding or whistling.
- Cosmetic change – Significant collapse (saddle nose) is rare, but subtle changes are probably under-recognised by patients and surgeons.

REFERENCES

1 Fettman N, Sanford T, Sindwani R (2009). Surgical management of the deviated septum: techniques in septoplasty. *Otolaryngologic Clinics of North America* **42**: 241–52, viii.
2 Goode RL, Smith LF (2nd edition 2001). Nasal septoplasty and submucous resection. In: Atlas of Head & Neck Surgery – Otolaryngology (pp. 462–4). Lippincott Williams & Wilkins, Philadelphia.
3 Moore M, Eccles R (2011). Objective evidence for the efficacy of surgical management of the deviated septum as treatment for chronic nasal obstruction: a systematic review. Clinical Otolaryngology doi: 10.1111/j.1749-4486.2011.02279.x [epub ahead of print].
4 Karatzanis AD, Fragiadakis G, Moshandrea J, *et al* (2009). Septoplasty outcome in patients with and without allergic rhinitis. *Rhinology* **47**: 444–9.
5 Gubisch W (2005). Extracorporeal septoplasty for the markedly deviated nasal septum. *Archives of Facial Plastic Surgery* **7**: 218–26.

6 Benjamin E, Wong DKK, Choa D (2004). 'Moffett's' solution: a review of the evidence and scientific basis for the topical preparation of the nose. *Clinical Otolaryngology* **29**: 582–7.

7 Paradis J, Rotenberg BW (2011). Open versus endoscopic septoplasty: a single-blinded, randomized, controlled trial. *Journal of Otolaryngology Head and Neck Surgery* **40** (Suppl. 1): S28–S33.

8 Jang YJ, Yeo NK, Wang JH (2009). Cutting and suture technique of the caudal septal cartilage for the management of caudal septal deviation. *Archives of Otolaryngology Head and Neck Surgery* **135**: 1256–60.

9 Kenyon GS, Kalan A, Jones NS (2002). Columelloplasty: a new suture technique to correct caudal septal cartilage dislocation. *Clinical Otolaryngology* **27**: 188–91.

10 SEPTORHINOPLASTY

There are numerous techniques involved in rhinoplasty surgery, which are beyond the scope of this book. Briefly, it can be divided into the endonasal (closed) approach and the external (open) approach (1). The endonasal approach is discussed here.

Indications

● Cosmetic correction of a deviated nose and septum. If there is severe deviation of the mid- and lower thirds of the nose, such as in the 'twisted nose', then an extracorporeal septoplasty technique may be required (2).

● Functional – To correct nasal obstruction that would not be successfully managed by simple septoplasty alone.

PREOPERATIVE REVIEW

Patient selection in rhinoplasty is paramount; their expectations must be realistic. Standard preoperative photographs are required in lateral, frontal, oblique, bird's eye and basal views.

OPERATIVE PROCEDURE

An appropriately informed, consented and anaesthetized patient is positioned supine, head up, with a head ring for support. Topical nasal preparations such as Moffett's solution (a variable mixture of cocaine, adrenaline, normal saline and sodium bicarbonate) (6) or co-phenylcaine spray (5% lidocaine, 0.5% phenylephrine) may be instilled into the nose to improve the surgical field. The patient's eyes are taped closed or lubricating ointment is instilled. A headlight is worn, although overhead operating lights may be used, particularly in the external approach.

Skin preparation is used around the nose. The patient is draped with a head towel so that the whole face is exposed.

The septum is infiltrated with 2% lidocaine with 1:80 000 adrenaline as for a septoplasty (Chapter 9). Infiltration is continued superiorly in the nasal vestibules along the lines of intercartilaginous incisions (Figure 10.1) and into the soft tissue overlying the dorsum of the nose, particularly at the incision sites for external lateral osteotomies. The nasal hairs are trimmed with short curved scissors.

Septoplasty is performed using a left hemitransfixion incision as described in Chapter 9. Once this is completed, bilateral intercartilaginous incisions are made between the upper and lower lateral cartilages. The groove between the cartilages is

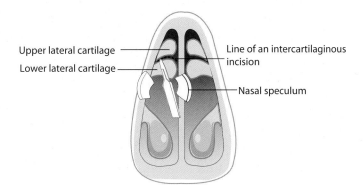

Figure 10.1. Intercartilaginous incision.

best displayed using an alar retractor with external pressure from the surgeon's middle finger. Care is taken not to incise the cartilages themselves. On the left the incision is continued caudally into the hemitransfixion incision. The hemitransfixion incision is extended to complete a full transfixion incision (through-and-through), although this does not need to extend completely to the base of the columella.

The dorsal and lateral nasal skin and soft tissue envelope is then degloved with a no. 15 scalpel blade or curved scissors, taking care not to button-hole the skin by staying on cartilage and bone. The skin is freed sufficiently to allow visualization of the nasal dorsum with an Aufricht's retractor and the scissors to pass freely from one side of the nose to the other. Release the procerus muscle at the nasion using a periosteal elevator.

If there is a dorsal hump, it can be removed with a 6–8 mm osteotome, taking care not to buttonhole the skin at either side (Figure 10.2). The dorsum is then rasped smooth.

Bilateral medial osteotomies are performed internally, using a 4–6 mm osteotome placed through the intercartilaginous incision. The osteotome is positioned perpendicular to the bone at the caudal end of the nasal bone, just lateral to the septum (3). The line of the osteotomy is shown in Figure 10.3. The assistant gently taps with a mallet, while the surgeon's palpates the edge of the osteotome to

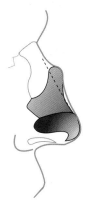

Figure 10.2. An osteotome may be used to remove a dorsal hump once the overlying soft tissue envelope has been lifted. The line of the osteotomy is illustrated.

ensure its position and to prevent buttonholing the skin. External lateral osteotomies are performed using a 2 mm osteotome via small stab incisions made with a no. 11 scalpel blade. The line of the osteotomy is 'scratched' onto the bone before being 'postage-stamped' where multiple small osteotomies are made along the lines shown in Figure 10.3. The assistant stabilizes the patient's head while the surgeon employs the mallet. Firm digital pressure is used to reposition the bones appropriately.

In more complex cases, tip work or grafts may be required; these are often better undertaken via an external approach.

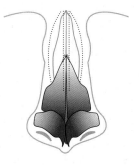

Figure 10.3. Medial and lateral osteotomy.

The incisions are closed with an absorbable suture. The same suture is used to 'quilt' the septum with through-and-through mattress sutures to reduce the risk of septal haematoma formation by closing the dead space, as for standard septoplasty. Steristrips are applied over the dorsum and to support the tip, and a triangular plaster of Paris is placed. Nasal packing is not routinely inserted.

POSTOPERATIVE REVIEW

The patient can be discharged with analgesia after observation according to the hospital's day surgery protocol. Patients are advised to have two weeks off work and to avoid heavy lifting or strenuous exercise, avoid nose-blowing for one week, and sneeze with their mouth open if possible. They are warned to expect periorbital bruising and swelling. Initial follow-up is after 5–7 days for removal of the plaster, after which patients can begin to douche the nose.

Complications

- Bleeding – Some oozing is normal but heavy epistaxis requires return to hospital and may warrant nasal packing. If a septal haematoma develops, it will require draining and packing.
- Infection.
- Ongoing obstructive symptoms – Either related to persistent/recurrent deviation as septal cartilage has 'memory', or to concurrent mucosal disease.

- Septal perforation – Usually asymptomatic, but may cause crusting, bleeding or whistling.
- Ongoing cosmetic concerns – Patients should be advised of a 5–10% revision rate following primary rhinoplasty surgery.

REFERENCES
1 Gillman GS (2008). Basic rhinoplasty. In: Operative Otolaryngology Head and Neck Surgery (pp. 806–10). Saunders, Philadelphia.
2 Senyuva C, Yücel A, Aydin Y, *et al* (1997). Extracorporeal septoplasty combined with open rhinoplasty. *Aesthetic Plastic Surgery* **21**: 233–39.
3 Calhoun KC (2nd edition 2001). Osteotomies. In: Atlas of Head & Neck Surgery – Otolaryngology (pp. 468–9). Lippincott Williams & Wilkins, Philadelphia.

11

TURBINATE SURGERY

Indications

● Nasal obstruction secondary to inferior turbinate hypertrophy refractory to medical treatment.

OPERATIVE PROCEDURE

There is an ever-increasing number of methods used to reduce inferior turbinate tissue and a recent Cochrane Review found no high-quality evidence for any technique (1). All are performed on an appropriately informed, consented and anaesthetized patient, positioned supine with a head ring for support, slightly head up. Topical nasal preparations such as Moffett's solution (a variable mixture of cocaine, adrenaline and sodium bicarbonate) (6) or co-phenylcaine spray (5% lidocaine, 0.5% phenylephrine) may be instilled into the nose to improve the surgical field. A headlight may be worn by the surgeon, or a rigid Hopkins rod used for endoscopic techniques. The patient's eyes are taped closed. Skin preparation is not routinely used. The patient is draped with a head towel.

▌ Out-fracture of the inferior turbinate

A Hill's elevator is used first to in-fracture the inferior turbinate (IT) and then out-fracture it (lateralize) (Figure 11.1).

▌ Submucous diathermy to the inferior turbinate

An insulated Thudichum's speculum is used to allow visualization of the IT. A monopolar diathermy Abbey needle is inserted into the inferior turbinate soft tissue, medial to the bone, along its full length. It is activated while being slowly withdrawn, cauterizing the erectile soft tissue. This is usually performed three times, superiorly, inferiorly and at the midpoint of the turbinate (Figure 11.2a and b).

A similar technique may be employed using two passes of a radiofrequency probe (2).

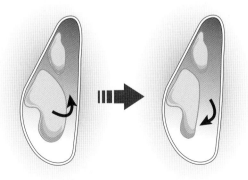

Figure 11.1. Out-fracture of the inferior turbinate.

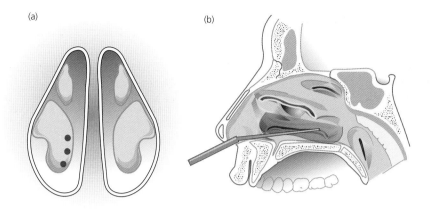

(a)   (b)

Figure 11.2. Submucous diathermy of the right inferior turbinate.

▌ Submucosal out-fracture of the inferior turbinate (SMOFIT)

The anterior end of the IT is infiltrated with 2% lidocaine with 1:80 000 adrenaline using a dental syringe. The IT is in-fractured as above, and a small stab incision is then made in the anterior end over the turbinate bone. A Freer's elevator is used to elevate the soft tissue off the turbinate bone along its full length. As it is withdrawn, the Freer's elevator is used to out-fracture the bone at multiple points along its length.

▌ Inferior turbinoplasty

There are multiple methods and instruments used to reduce the IT soft tissue. Following a SMOFIT (as above), a small Tilley Henkel forceps can be used to remove pieces of bone and soft tissue. This can be done endoscopically for more controlled reduction. A laser may be used, and a turbinoplasty microdebrider attachment is also available, which is inserted through a stab incision as above and allows powered removal of IT bone and soft tissue (3).

▌ Turbinectomy

This may be performed using a headlight or endoscope. The IT is in-fractured as above, then

turbinectomy scissors are used to trim its inferomedial aspect (Figure 11.3).

A small dressing (e.g., ribbon gauze soaked in adrenaline, or a piece of non-adhesive gauze) may be left in the nose during the recovery period. If there is significant bleeding, a nasal tampon may be required, in which case the patient is kept in overnight and the pack removed the following morning.

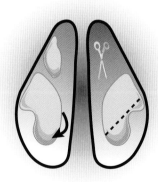

Figure 11.3. Turbinectomy. Care must be taken to avoid damage to the nasolacrimal duct.

POSTOPERATIVE REVIEW

Any small pack may be removed after 1–2 hours. The patient can be discharged after observation according to the hospital's day surgery protocol. Discharge medication includes analgesia and nasal douches; regular intranasal treatment for rhinitis should be recommenced after a few days. Patients are advised to take one week off work, avoid nose-blowing for one week, sneeze with their mouth open if possible and avoid heavy lifting or strenuous exercise for two weeks. Follow-up may be arranged.

Complications

- Bleeding – This may be profuse and patients should be warned of the potential need for a blood transfusion. The risk is higher with turbinectomy than the turbinoplasty procedures.
- Nasal crusting – Turbinectomy leaves a large raw area, unlike turbinoplasty; diathermy can also cause crusting.
- Adhesions – Between the IT and septum.
- Empty nose syndrome – Excessive removal of IT tissue causes worsening symptoms of obstruction due to loss of sensation of nasal airflow, hence the newer turbinoplasty procedures do not remove turbinate mucosa.
- Ongoing/recurrent symptoms – Any benefit may be temporary and ongoing medical treatment of rhinitis may be required postoperatively.

REFERENCES

1 Jose J, Coatesworth AP (2010). Inferior turbinate surgery for nasal obstruction in allergic rhinitis after failed medical management. Cochrane Database of Systematic Reviews 8: CD005235.
2 Cavaliere M, Mottola G, Iemma M (2005). Comparison of the effectiveness and safety of radiofrequency turbinoplasty and traditional surgical technique in the treatment of inferior turbinate hypertrophy. *Otolaryngology Head and Neck Surgery* **133**: 972–8.
3 Lee DH, Kim EH (2010). Microdebrider-assisted versus laser-assisted turbinate reduction: comparison of improvement in nasal airway according to type of turbinate hypertrophy. *Ear Nose and Throat Journal* **89**: 541–5.

12 ANTRAL WASHOUT

This procedure is rarely performed as it has been almost completely superseded by endoscopic sinus surgery (1). It is now generally reserved for the sick patient unfit for formal endoscopic sinus surgery in whom the maxillary sinus is thought to harbour infection and when cultures are required. This procedure can be performed under local anaesthetic on the intensive care unit if necessary.

Indications

● Acute maxillary sinusitis unresponsive to medical treatment.
● To provide diagnostic cultures.

OPERATIVE PROCEDURE

An appropriately informed, consented and anaesthetized patient (where possible) should be positioned head up with a head ring for support. If the patient is sedated or under general anaesthesia, topical nasal preparations such as Moffett's solution (a variable mixture of cocaine, adrenaline and sodium bicarbonate) or co-phenylcaine spray (5% lidocaine, 0.5% phenylephrine) may be instilled into the nose to improve the surgical field. If the patient is awake, 2% lidocaine with 1:80 000 adrenaline may be infiltrated into the lateral nasal wall adjacent to the inferior turbinate (IT). A headlight is worn and the nasal cavity examined using a nasal speculum.

The IT is in-fractured (medialized) using a Hill's or Freer's elevator and a sheathed antral washout trocar is passed into the nasal cavity. The trocar is inserted beneath the IT, approximately 1.5–2 cm posterior to its anterior attachment (to avoid damage to the nasolacrimal duct). The trocar is aimed laterally, in the direction of the ipsilateral tragus (Figure 12.1).

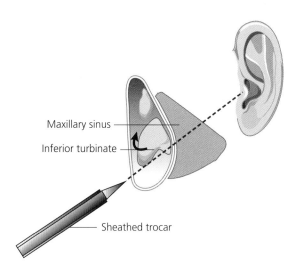

Maxillary sinus

Inferior turbinate

Sheathed trocar

Figure 12.1. Antral washout. Once in-fractured, a sheathed trocar is inserted beneath the inferior turbinate. Gentle force is used to direct the tip of the trocar towards the external auditory canal of the ipsilateral ear.

The needle is gently advanced while the eye is held open by an assistant (a misplaced trocar may enter the orbital cavity). A 'give' is often felt as the trocar enters the antrum.

Once in place, the trocar is withdrawn, leaving the sheath *in situ*. The maxillary sinus may be irrigated with a 20 mL syringe of saline. Fluid can then be aspirated to provide a sample for culture. Irrigation is continued until the aspirate is clear. It is essential to watch the patient's eye carefully during irrigation to ensure the sheath is not within the orbit.

Nasal packing is not routinely required.

Complications

- Bleeding.
- Nasolacrimal duct injury.
- Subcutaneous emphysema due to misplacement of the trocar superficial to the antrum.
- Orbital injury due to misplacement of trocar; this technique is contraindicated in patients with a hypoplastic maxillary sinus as this risk is increased.

REFERENCES

1 Lazar RH, Mitchell RB (2nd edition 2001). Intranasal antrostomy through the inferior meatus. In: Atlas of Head & Neck Surgery – Otolaryngology (pp. 916–17). Lippincott Williams & Wilkins, Philadelphia.

13 ENDOSCOPIC SINUS SURGERY

Also referred to as functional endoscopic sinus surgery (FESS), the aim of endoscopic sinus surgery (ESS) is to improve the drainage and function of the paranasal sinuses. Mucosal stripping is to be avoided and the natural sinus ostia are opened whenever possible. There are a number of extended applications for ESS, including those listed below (1).

Indications

● Chronic rhinosinusitis with or without nasal polyps, refractory to maximum medical treatment.

● Recurrent acute sinusitis.
● Complications of acute sinusitis that have failed medical management.
● Sinus mucocoeles.
● Sinonasal tumour excision.
● Endoscopic dacrocystorhinostomy (DCR).
● Orbital or optic nerve decompression.
● Endoscopic repair of CSF leak.
● Transphenoidal approach to the pituitary/anterior skull base lesions.

PREOPERATIVE REVIEW

A CT scan of the sinuses is mandatory and should be available at the time of surgery. This must be reviewed preoperatively by the surgeon to evaluate the extent of disease, any previous surgery or bony loss and any anatomical variants (1).

OPERATIVE PROCEDURE

An appropriately informed, consented and anaesthetized patient should be positioned supine with a head ring for support, slightly head up. Topical nasal preparations such as Moffett's solution (a variable mixture of cocaine, adrenaline and sodium bicarbonate) or co-phenylcaine spray (5% lidocaine, 0.5% phenylephrine) are instilled into the nose to improve the surgical field. The patient's eyes are not taped or covered, but lubricating ointment is instilled. This allows immediate identification of any orbital bleeding, and the eye to be balloted, while observing the lateral nasal wall for any evidence of movement (suggesting a dehiscent lamina papyracea). Skin preparation is not routinely used. The patient is draped with a head towel.

A 0° rigid Hopkins rod endoscope is used to inspect the nasal cavities bilaterally using the three-pass technique (see Chapter 2). The first pass is along the floor of the nose to the postnasal space, assessing the inferior meatus (Figure 13.1). The second is into the middle meatus, and the third into the superior meatus and olfactory niche; the sphenoid ostium may be identified during this pass. Important landmarks to note are the septum, inferior and middle turbinates and the posterior choana (Figure 13.2).

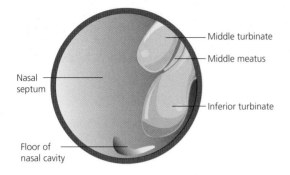

Figure 13.1. First pass along the floor of the nose (left nasal cavity).

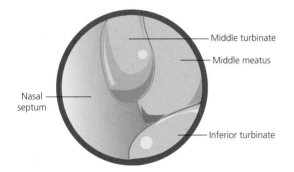

Figure 13.2. The second pass allows access to the middle meatus.

At this point, it is often helpful to insert adrenaline-soaked neuropatties or ribbon gauze into the middle meatus, using a Freer's elevator for accurate positioning. This provides further decongestion and vasoconstriction to improve the surgical field.

The middle turbinate should not be forcefully medialized as this risks skull base fracture with CSF leak. It can be gently moved out of the way of instruments, but if very large and obstructing, then a wedge can be removed from the anterior end with a through-cutting punch, whilst preserving the majority as an anatomical landmark (Figure 13.3).

The uncinate process is palpated with the Freer's elevator (Figure 13.4).

A Freer's elevator or a sickle knife is used to perform an uncinectomy and expose the natural ostium of the maxillary sinus. Incise along the anterior attachment of the uncinate process from superior to inferior (Figure 13.5). Care should be taken not to enter the orbit with this incision.

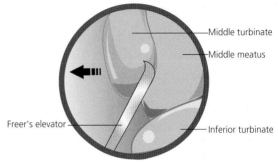

Figure 13.3. Gentle mediatization of the middle turbinate to access to the middle meatus.

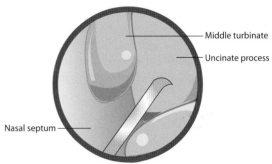

Figure 13.4. Palpation of the uncinate process with a Freer's elevator.

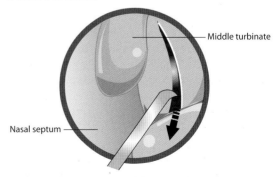

Figure 13.5. Incision along the anterior attachment of the uncinate process.

The uncinate process will become apparent as a sickle-shaped thin sheet of bone with a free posterior edge. Small scissors may be used to cut through the remaining superior and inferior attachments of the uncinate process, or straight Blakesley-Wilde forceps can be used directly to remove it with a twisting motion to avoid tearing the mucosa (Figure 13.6).

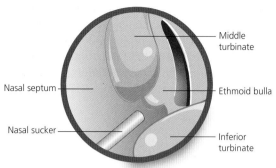

Figure 13.7. Opening of the ethmoid bulla.

The anterior ethmoids are opened with a curette or Blakesley-Wilde forceps, as may the posterior ethmoids if indicated (Figure 13.8). Appropriately trained and experienced surgeons may perform sphenoid sinus and frontal recess surgery, as required.

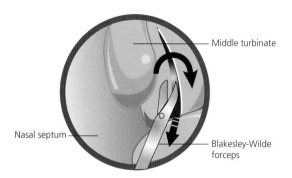

Figure 13.6. Removal of the uncinate process.

The uncinate process may also be removed using a retrograde technique with backbiting forceps placed behind the free posterior edge of the uncinate process. This is thought to reduce the risk of orbital penetration (2).

Once the uncinectomy is complete, the natural maxillary ostium should be visible and the ethmoid bulla will also now be in view (Figure 13.7).

A curved sucker may be passed into the sinus to remove any mucus or pus. The antrostomy may be widened if necessary using a backbiting forceps. The bulla can be opened using straight or 45°-angled Blakesley-Wilde forceps or a sucker as illustrated in Figure 13.7.

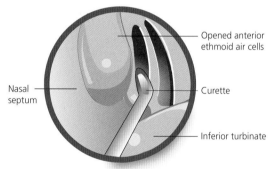

Figure 13.8. Opening of the anterior ethmoids.

If bleeding is minimal, then no packing is required. Depending on the surgeon's preference and the amount of bleeding, packing may be inserted in the form of adrenaline-soaked ribbon gauze, non-adhesive gauze, nasal tampon or newer absorbable packing materials.

POSTOPERATIVE REVIEW

If nasal packing is inserted, it can be removed in recovery, on the ward or the next morning, depending on the amount of oozing. The patient may be discharged after observation according to the hospi-

tal's day surgery protocol, or may require overnight admission. Discharge medication can include analgesia, oral and/or topical nasal steroids and nasal douches. Antibiotics may be given, often depending on an intraoperative finding of infection. Patients are advised to avoid nose-blowing for one week, sneeze with their mouth open if possible and have 10–14 days off work while avoiding heavy lifting or strenuous exercise during this period. If follow-up is planned, this should be after two weeks to allow for outpatient decrusting of the nasal cavities.

Complications

- Bleeding – Some oozing is normal but heavy epistaxis requires return to hospital and may warrant nasal packing or rarely return to theatre. Perioperative haemorrhage occurs in approximately 5% of cases, with significant postoperative bleeding in less than 1% (3).
- Infection.
- Nasal crusting – Minimized with regular douching and early outpatient review.
- Adhesions – Usually between the middle turbinate and the lateral nasal wall, but can occur between the inferior turbinate and the septum if traumatized during surgery.
- Recurrent symptoms – In certain cases (e.g., chronic rhinosinusitis with or without nasal polyps) it is important to make patients aware that ESS may not be a cure for the underlying disease process and that symptoms can recur. Patients are therefore advised to continue long-term treatment with intranasal steroids and douche after surgery.
- Orbital injury or bleeding – Occurs in approximately 0.2% of cases (3).
- CSF leak – Occurs in approximately 0.06% of cases (3).

REFERENCES

1 Wormald P-J (2005). Endoscopic Sinus Surgery: Anatomy, Three-Dimensional Reconstruction, and Surgical Technique. Thieme Medical Publishers, New York.
2 Schaitkin BM (2008). Maxillary sinus: the endoscopic approach. In: Operative Otolaryngology Head and Neck Surgery (pp. 53–4). Saunders, Philadelphia.
3 Hopkins C, Browne JP, Slack R, et al (2006). Complication of surgery for nasal polyposis and chronic rhinosinusitis: the results of a national audit in England and Wales. *Laryngoscope* **116**: 1494–9.

14 NASAL POLYPECTOMY

Indications

- Nasal polyposis causing obstructive symptoms despite maximum medical management.

- Histological identification in cases of unilateral polyps.

PREOPERATIVE REVIEW

As nasal polypectomy is now invariably performed as an endoscopic procedure, a CT scan of the sinuses is mandatory. This must be available at the time of surgery and reviewed preoperatively by the surgeon to evaluate the extent of disease, any previous surgery or bony loss and anatomical variants. Nasal polypectomy is commonly combined with endoscopic sinus surgery (ESS), as there is evidence that even limited ESS can reduce revision rates over a five-year period (1).

OPERATIVE PROCEDURE

An appropriately informed, consented and anaesthetized patient is positioned supine with a head ring for support, slightly head up. Topical nasal preparations such as Moffett's solution (a variable mixture of cocaine, adrenaline and sodium bicarbonate) or co-phenylcaine spray (5% lidocaine, 0.5% phenylephrine) are instilled into the nose to improve the surgical field. The patient's eyes are not taped or covered, but lubricating ointment is instilled to allow immediate identification of any orbital bleeding. Skin preparation is not routinely used. The patient is draped with a head towel.

A 0° rigid Hopkins rod endoscope is used to inspect the nasal cavities. Representative biopsies are taken from both sides, particularly if a microdebrider is to be used. Short pieces of ribbon gauze or neurosurgical patties soaked in adrenaline are inserted bilaterally for vasoconstriction.

Various methods are available, but the two most commonly used are:

1 Direct removal with grasping instruments such as Tilley Henkels or Blakesley-Wilde forceps; 45°-angled forceps may be useful for more complete clearance superiorly. Care must be taken not to exert too much force when removing tissue; gentle pressure or a twisting motion should be sufficient.
2 Powered instrumentation in the form of a microdebrider. This instrument consists of an oscillating cutting blade within a sheath, attached to irrigation and suction. Care must be taken to ensure that the tip of the instrument can be seen at all times to avoid damage to adjacent structures.

Ideally all polyps are removed. If bleeding is minimal, then no packing is required. Depending on the surgeon's preference and the amount of bleeding, packing may be inserted in the form of adrenaline-soaked ribbon gauze, non-adhesive gauze, nasal tampon or newer absorbable packing materials.

POSTOPERATIVE REVIEW

If nasal packing is inserted, it can be removed in recovery, on the ward or the next morning depending on the degree of oozing. The patient may be discharged after observation according to the hospital's day surgery protocol, or may require overnight admission. Discharge medication can include analgesia, oral and/or topical nasal steroids and nasal douches. Antibiotics may be given, depending on the intraoperative finding of infection. Patients are advised to take 10–14 days off work and to avoid heavy lifting or strenuous exercise during this period. They should avoid nose-blowing for one week and sneeze with their mouth open if possible.

Complications

- Bleeding – Some oozing is normal but heavy epistaxis requires return to hospital and may warrant nasal packing or rarely return to theatre.
- Infection.
- Recurrent polyps – It is important to make patients aware that polypectomy is not a cure for the underlying disease process and that polyps tend to recur. They are therefore advised to continue long-term treatment with intranasal steroids and douche after surgery.
- Persistent anosmia – Surgical polypectomy does not guarantee the return of a sense of smell and may even reduce it.
- Orbital injury or bleeding – Unlikely in the absence of formal ESS but the lamina papyracea may be dehiscent in nasal polyposis.
- CSF leak – Unlikely in the absence of formal ESS but polyps removal in the region of the olfactory niche may damage the cribriform plate.

REFERENCE

1 Hopkins C, Slack R, Lund V, et al (2009). Long-term outcomes from the English national comparative audit of surgery for nasal polyposis and chronic rhinosinusitis. *Laryngoscope* **119**: 2459–65.

15 TYMPANOPLASTY

DEFINITION

Tympanoplasty is the term used for the surgical eradication of middle ear disease and the restoration of middle ear function, including the reconstruction of the tympanic membrane and ossicular chain (ossiculoplasty).

Historically, Wullstein described five types of tympanoplasty (1):

Type 1   Myringoplasty – Closure of a tympanic membrane perforation.
Type 2   Reconstruction of the tympanic membrane over the malleus remnant and long process of incus.
Type 3   Reconstruction of the tympanic membrane over the head of the stapes.
Type 4   Reconstruction of the tympanic membrane over the round window.
Type 5   Reconstruction of the tympanic membrane over an artificial fenestration in the basal turn of the cochlea.
Type 6   Reconstruction of the tympanic membrane over an artificial fenestration in the horizontal semicircular canal.

Only two of these remain relevant today.

Type I tympanoplasty describes the reconstruction of the tympanic membrane in the presence of an intact and mobile ossicular chain. This procedure is synonymous with the term myringoplasty.

Type III tympanoplasty describes the reconstruction performed when the incus and malleus have been removed or eroded by disease. The tympanic membrane is reconstructed to lie on the stapes head to create a columella effect or myringostapedopexy. The same principle is applied with some ossiculoplasty procedures where the stapes superstructure or footplate is in contact with the reconstructed tympanic membrane via a prosthesis.

Indications

● Recurrent ear infection.
● Hearing loss.
● To 'waterproof' the ear.

The main indications for tympanoplasty are chronic secretory otitis media, either mucosal (tympanic membrane perforation) or with cholesteatoma, and the surgical management of pars tensa retraction pockets (Figure 15.1). These conditions often result in ear discharge (otorrhoea), conductive hearing loss and the social inconvenience of being unable to get the ear wet.

PRE-OPERATIVE ASSESSMENT

▌ History

Establish the nature of the symptoms and the impact these have on the patients; quality of life; this will help when counseling them. Does the ear discharge? How often? Is it painful? Is there any subjective hearing loss? Is there any associated vertigo or tinnitus? What about the other ear? Is there any other relevant ENT history?

▌ Examination

Document the position (central or marginal) and size of the perforation. Is there an associated cholesteatoma? Describe the status of the middle ear (dry or infected). Is it possible to comment on the state of the ossicular chain? If there is a pars tensa retraction pocket, it is helpful to use the descriptive Sade classification (See Table 15.1). Document the state of the contralateral ear.

Table 15.1. Sade classification (2).

Grade	Description
1	Mild retraction of pars tensa
2	Retraction touching the incus or stapes
3	Retraction touching the promontory
4	Tympanic membrane adherent to the promontory

▌ Investigations

Pure tone audiometry, including air conduction and appropriately masked bone conduction, is an essential part of the assessment and should be performed within three months of surgery.

Imaging of the temporal bone is not usually required for a simple perforation. If there is cholesteatoma and a concurrent mastoidectomy procedure is planned, a high resolution fine-cut CT scan of the temporal bones is recommended to act as a 'roadmap' for surgery.

MYRINGOPLASTY

▌ Aims of surgery

The principal aims of surgery are to provide the patient with an intact tympanic membrane resulting in a safe and dry ear that hears as well as possible.

▌ Alternatives to surgery

In addition to discussing surgery, it is important to advise patients of the alternatives available to them. In the case of a central perforation, these include observation coupled with water precautions, particularly if there are few symptoms and the impact on lifestyle is minimal. A trial of a hearing aid is an option if hearing loss is the primary symptom.

Complications

- Scar (potential for poor cosmesis).
- Bleeding.
- Infection.
- Graft failure (personal audit will determine this risk – 10–30%).
- Chorda tympani injury with taste disturbance (usually temporary).
- Ear numbness (particularly with a post-auricular incision).
- Hearing loss (dead ear <1%).
- Tinnitus (rare).
- Vertigo (rare).
- Facial nerve palsy (usually temporary and rare).

OPERATIVE PROCEDURE

Preoperatively, it is important to ensure the patient is adequately marked, has an up-to-date audiogram and still has the perforation (Figure 15.1a).

Do not assume that the anaesthetist is familiar with the type of surgery planned. In particular, discuss the need for intraoperative hypotension to reduce bleeding and lack of paralysis to enable facial nerve monitoring.

The patient is placed supine, with their head on a head ring, rotated away from the operative ear. A small amount of hair removal may be required. We recommend the use of a facial nerve monitor as if it is used for all otological cases (other than insertion of a grommet), then the entire theatre team become familiar with how to set it up and there is no ambiguity as to whether it is required for a particular procedure. It is also useful in the event of any unexpected pathology. Strapping the patient to the table is helpful and allows them to be rotated during surgery, which can improve visualization of middle ear structures. A useful check list prior to scrubbing up is to consider three S's:

- Side – correct side?
- Spikes (facial nerve monitor).
- Straps – is the patient secured to the table?

▌ Procedure steps

Injection of local anaesthetic

The use of a local anaesthetic such as 2% xylociane with 1:80 000 adrenaline is used to aid vasoconstriction. The procedure can be performed under local anaesthetic, but general anaesthesia is more common. The ear canal skin is infiltrated with local anaesthetic providing hydrodissection, making it easier to dissect and less likely to bleed. The site of any intended external incision is then infiltrated.

Remove margins of the perforation

With the perforation clearly in view a gently curved needle can be used to make a series of tiny perforations around it (Figure 15.1b). It is helpful to start inferiorly and work superiorly to prevent bleeding from the edge obscuring the view. The small perforations are joined together and, the inner ring

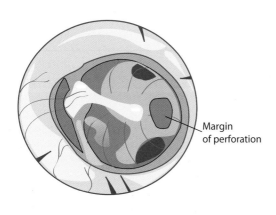

(a)

Figure 15.1. (a) Tympanic membrane perforation.

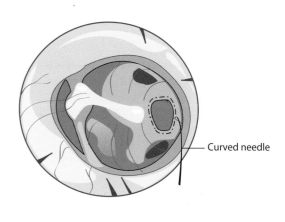

(b)

Figure 15.1. (b) Freshening the edge of the perforation.

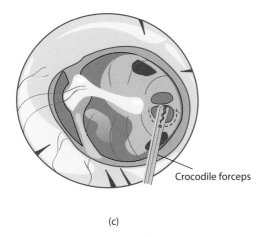

(c)

Figure 15.1. (c) Freshening edge of perforation.

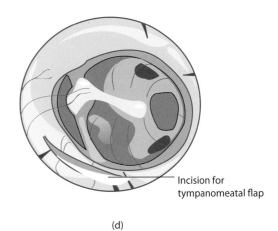

Incision for
tympanomeatal flap

(d)

Figure 15.1. (d) Tympanomeatal flap incision.

of tissue can be gently pulled away using crocodile or cupped forceps leaving a freshened and slightly larger perforation (Figure 15.1c).

Incision

There are three standard approaches for performing otological procedures. The choice usually comes down to surgeon preference. Adequate exposure of the entire perforation is essential and will influence which approach is used. It may also be necessary to perform a limited canalplasty to remove any bone obscuring the view of the perforation, particularly if there is an anterior canal wall overhang obscuring an anterior perforation.

- Permeatal – if the external auditory canal (EAC) permits a view of the entire perforation and is wide enough to accommodate a large speculum, this approach can be used for both small and large perforations. It is helpful to use as wide a speculum as the EAC will allow. This can be secured with a clear plastic drape.
- Post-auricular – a curved incision is made approximately 1 cm behind the post-auricular crease through the skin and subcutaneous tissue onto the temporalis fascia in its upper half. A semicircular incision is made through the periosteum just posterior to the bony EAC. The skin of the posterior EAC is then elevated prior to making a re-entry incision into the EAC (Figure 15.1d).

Tapes passed through the ear canal and out via the re-entry incision can be used to retract the pinna and lateral meatal skin out of the field of view.
- Pre-auricular (endaural) – an incision is made just anterior to the anterior helix of the pinna and runs inferiorly between the helix and tragus. It is continued into the roof of the EAC. A limb can be extended down the posterior wall of the EAC. The meatal skin lateral to this limb can then be elevated laterally over the bony margin of the ear canal. A two-prong retractor is then used to give exposure.

Tympanomeatal flap

Whatever approach is used, it is usually necessary to elevate a tympanomeatal flap, except in the cases of very small perforations, where a fat or facial graft can be 'tucked' through the perforation. A posteriorly placed bucket handle incision is made, extending from the 12 o'clock position of the tympanic membrane (TM) (adjacent to the lateral process of the handle of malleus) to beyond the 6 o'clock position. Microscissors are required for the thicker meatal skin of the superior EAC. The flap is elevated using an elevator such as a Rosen ring until the annulus is reached. A fine elevator such as a Hugh's is used to elevate the annulus and enter the middle ear. By entering the middle ear posteroinferiorly, injury to the chorda tympani is minimized. Once the TM is reflected anteriorly, it should be possible to see the medial surface of the anterior extent of the perforation. For a larger perforation, it is helpful to elevate the TM off the handle of malleus. An ophthalmic keratome knife is extremely useful for dividing the adherent fibres attaching the TM to the umbo.

Check the ossicular chain

Visually inspect the ossicles, in particular the incudostapedial joint (ISJ). Gently palpate the malleus handle and observe the movement of the malleus and incus (limited if there is attic fixation), confirm the integrity of the ISJ and mobility of the stapes footplate.

Graft harvest

The two commonest graft materials used are temporalis fascia and a composite cartilage perichondrium graft. Temporalis fascia is simply harvested via a post- or pre-auricular incision. To enable it to be easier to manipulate, it is scraped flat and left to dry. Cartilage can be harvested from the concha cymba, concha cavum or fossa triangularis if using a post-auricular incision or from the tragus if performing a permeatal or end-aural approach. The composite perichondrium cartilage graft technique uses a single shield or island-shaped graft that remains attached to its perichondrium to reconstruct part or all of the tympanic membrane. Cartilage composite grafts

have a very high success rate for repair of both small and large perforations, and are resilient to retraction without adversely affecting hearing outcomes (3).

Graft sizing

A helpful technique is to cut a paper template to accurately size the perforation or region of tympanic membrane that requires reconstruction. If using fascia, the graft will need to be bigger than the template. If using a composite island graft, the cartilage can be trimmed to the size of the perforation, while retaining a perichondrial apron to aid with graft placement.

Graft placement

The graft is placed beneath the tympanic membrane in an underlay fashion (Figure 15.1e) and manipulated such that the entire TM defect is sealed (Figure 15.1f). The graft should lie flat against the undersurface of the TM. Surface tension is usually adequate to keep the graft in place, but additional support can be obtained by placing small Gelfoam™ or Spongostan™ pieces in the middle ear. The tympanomeatal flap is then relocated in its original position.

Ear packing

The surface of the tympanic membrane is gently covered to protect it and allow epithelium to grow

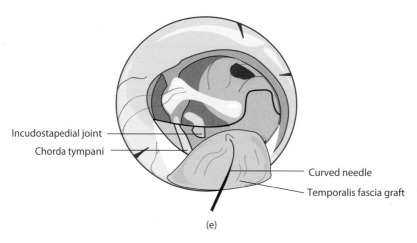

Incudostapedial joint
Chorda tympani
Curved needle
Temporalis fascia graft

(e)

Figure 15.1. (e) Underlay graft.

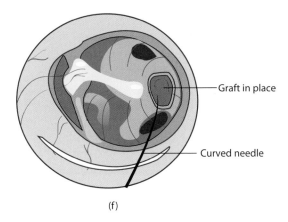

Graft in place

Curved needle

(f)

Figure 15.1. (f) Graft positioning.

over the graft. The dressing used is dependent on the preference of the surgeon. This can be done with a thin strip of clear silastic, small pieces of BIPP ribbon gauze or with gel foam blocks. The external auditory canal is then filled with further short strips of BIPP ribbon gauze (or similar) or a Pope wick in order to keep the meatal skin in place and prevent blunting of the angle between the TM and ear canal.

Closure

The wounds are closed in layers, preferably with an absorbable suture such as 4/0 Vicryl or Monocryl. A head bandage may or may not be required (four hours is usually adequate).

POSTOPERATIVE REVIEW

Postoperatively, it is good practice to document the facial nerve function and confirm that there is still hearing in the operated ear by performing a Weber test. The majority of myringoplasty cases can be performed as day surgery, particularly if performed permeatally.

Advise the patient to keep the ear dry until after review. Postoperative follow-up is usually 2–4 weeks after surgery, at which time the dressings are removed from the ear.

KEY POINTS:

- Audiometry – Ensure the patient has an up-to-date, ear-specific, appropriately masked audiogram prior to surgery.
- CT scan – A high-resolution temporal bone CT scan provides a useful 'roadmap' for mastoid surgery.
- Facial nerve monitor – Make it a routine part of your practice.
- Correct side.
- Optimal access and visualization. The local anaesthetic, hypotensive general anaesthetic, surgical approach and ability to manoeuvre the operating table combine to provide the best surgical conditions.

REFERENCES

1 Wullstein H (1956). Theory and practice of tympanoplasty. *Laryngoscope* **66**: 1976–93.
2 Sade J, Berco E (1976). Atelectasis and secretory otis media. *American Journal of Otolaryngology* **85**(Suppl. 25): 66–72.
3 Dornhoffer J (2003). Cartilage tympanoplasty: indications, techniques and outcomes in a 1000 patient series. *Laryngoscope* **113**(11): 1844–56.

16 MASTOIDECTOMY

Mastoidectomy is the surgical removal of all or part of the petromastoid portion of the temporal bone. The degree of removal depends on the condition being addressed.

Indications

- For pathology – Removal of disease within the mastoid air cells or from the middle ear, including acute mastoiditis, malignancy, mucosal chronic secretory otitis media (CSOM) and, most commonly, CSOM with cholesteatoma.
- For access – The mastoid component of the temporal bone acts as a conduit for a number of surgical procedures, including hearing implantation surgery (cochlear and middle ear), endolymphatic sac surgery, labyrinth surgery (posterior or superior semicircular canal occlusion and osseous labyrinthectomy) and translabyrinthine approaches to the internal auditory canal and cerebellopontine angle (vestibular schwannoma surgery).

CHOLESTEATOMA SURGERY

Cholesteatoma is keratinizing squamous epithelium (skin cells) within the middle ear space. They tend to gradually enlarge. The combination of enzyme production and pressure necrosis can result in the destruction of bony structures, including the ossicles and otic capsule.

ASSESSMENT

▌ History

Cholesteatomas present with a painless discharging ear (often with an unpleasant odour) and an associated hearing loss. Less commonly, they can present with one of the more serious complications of CSOM with cholesteatoma, including meningitis, acute mastoiditis, facial nerve palsy and vertigo secondary to a lateral semicircular canal fistula. As with any otological procedure, the condition of the contralateral ear is an important consideration.

▌ Examination

Document the origin of the cholesteatoma. Does it originate in the attic, from a marginal perforation or pars tensa retraction pocket? Describe the status of the middle ear (dry or infected?), including the state of the ossicular chain. Document the state of the contralateral ear.

▌ Investigations

Pure tone audiometry, including air conduction and appropriately masked bone conduction, is an essential part of the assessment and should be performed within three months of surgery.

An axial high-resolution fine-cut CT scan of the temporal bones with coronal reconstructions is an important component of management. This is not performed for diagnostic purposes, which is clinical, but serves as a 'roadmap' for planning surgery to determine:

- The extent of cholesteatoma (often unreliable).
- Whether the sigmoid sinus is dominant or situated anteriorly.
- The level of the middle fossa dura and whether this is dehiscent.

- The course of the facial nerve and whether this is dehiscent.
- Whether there is erosion of the otic capsule.
- The state of the ossicles.

A number of different mastoidectomy techniques can be employed in the treatment of cholesteatoma (Figure 16.1a). These include:

- Combined approach tympanoplasty (CAT), also known as a canal wall up mastoidectomy (Figure 16.1b).
- Atticotomy or small cavity mastoidectomy, also known as front-to-back mastoidectomy.
- Modified radical mastoidectomy, also known as a canal wall down mastoidectomy (Figure 16.1c).

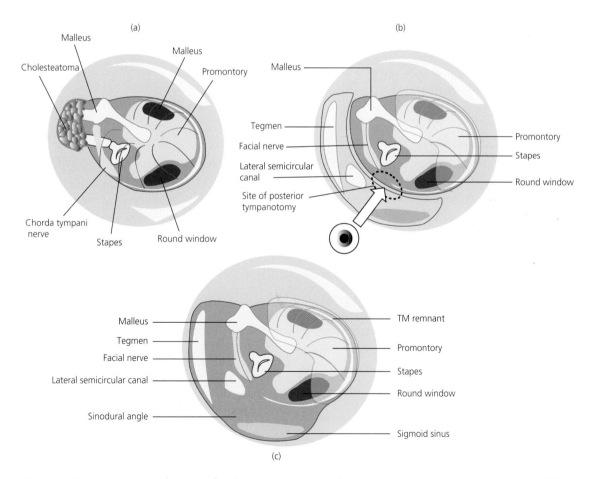

Figure 16.1. (a–c) Surgical options for cholesteatoma (a) include combined approach tympanoplasty (b) or modified radical mastoidectomy (c).

A good otologist should be trained in all three techniques so that the procedure performed can be tailored to the specific disease and requirements of the patient.

AIMS OF SURGERY

The principal aims of surgery are to provide the patient with a safe, dry ear that hears to the best of its ability and to eradicate the risks associated with untreated cholesteatoma.

ALTERNATIVES TO SURGERY

When discussing surgery, it is important to advise patients of the alternatives available to them. In the case of cholesteatoma, surgery is the only means of eradicating the disease and the associated complications. Observation is an option in selected cases, in particular, in patients who are symptom-free, too unfit for surgery or who decline surgery.

Cholesteatoma in an only hearing ear is not an absolute contraindication to surgery, but it is advisable that any procedure is undertaken by an experienced otologist.

■ Complications

The risks of surgery include:

● Scar (potential for poor cosmesis).
● Bleeding.

● Infection.
● Residual or recurrent disease (up to 25% with CAT, hence the need for second-look surgery).
● Facial nerve injury (<1%).
● Chorda tympani injury with taste disturbance (usually temporary even if the chorda is divided).
● Ear numbness (particularly with post-auricular incision).
● Hearing loss (risk of dead ear up to 1%).
● Tinnitus (rare).
● Vertigo (rare).

OPERATION

Preoperatively, it is important to ensure the patient is adequately marked and has an up-to-date audiogram. Review the CT scan and determine whether any complicating factors are anticipated.

Check the availability of any specialist equipment with the scrub team. This may include an adequate selection of the preferred ossicular replacement prostheses, the availability of a KTP laser with appropriately trained operator or a range of otoendoscopes.

Ensure that the anaesthetist is aware of the need for intraoperative facial nerve monitoring and relative hypotension to reduce bleeding.

The patient is placed supine, with their head on a head ring, rotated away from the operative ear. A small amount of peri-auricular hair removal may be required. Most otologists regard the use of a facial nerve monitor for cholesteatoma surgery as mandatory if the hospital is in possession of the device. Strapping the patient to the table is extremely helpful and allows them to be rotated during surgery to improve visualization of difficult areas. Many surgeons mark the planned postaural incision and mastoid process (Figure 16.2a). A useful checklist prior to scrubbing up is to consider three S's:

- Side – Correct side?
- Spikes – Facial nerve monitor.
- Straps – Is the patient secured to the table?

▌ Combined Approach Tympanoplasty

Procedure steps

1 Injection of local anaesthetic – The use of a local anaesthetic such as 2% xylociane with 1:80 000 adrenaline is used to infiltrate the canal skin and the region of the post-auricular incision (Figure 16.2b).

2 Incision (post-auricular) – A curved incision is made 1–2 cm behind the post-auricular crease through skin and subcutaneous tissue onto temporalis fascia in its upper half (Figure 16.2c). A horseshoe incision is made through the periosteum of the mastoid and a superiorly based subperiosteal flap raised (Figure 16.2d–e) using a periosteal elevator (Figure 16.2f). The skin of the posterior EAC is then elevated prior to making a re-entry incision into the EAC. Tapes passed through the ear canal and out via the re-entry incision are used to keep the pinna and lateral meatal skin retracted. This approach provides excellent exposure of the cortical bone of the mastoid and the root of the zygomatic process.

3 Tympanomeatal flap and disease isolation – The goal is to isolate the middle ear component of the cholesteatoma, while preserving the healthy remnant of the tympanic membrane. As with a myringoplasty, a posteriorly placed bucket handle incision is made, extending from the 12 o'clock position of the TM (adjacent to the lateral process of the handle of malleus) to beyond the 6 o'clock position. The superior aspect of the tympanomeatal flap incision is taken right up to the margin of cholesteatoma. Microscissors are used to cut around the neck of the cholesteatoma. It may be necessary to divide the chorda tympani cleanly if it is involved in the disease. The resulting flap of posterior canal skin and tympanic membrane remnant is elevated and reflected anteroinferiorly. At the same time, the TM may be elevated off the handle of malleus. An ophthalmic keratome knife is useful for dividing the adherent fibres attaching the TM to the umbo.

4 Check the ossicular chain – Visually inspect the ossicles and their relationship with the cholesteatoma. If the ossicular chain is intact, a decision regarding whether it will be possible to clear disease adequately without disrupting it must be made. With a more extensive cholesteatoma involving the mesotympanum, it may be necessary to remove disease in order to get a view of the incus and or stapes. In these cases, there is often erosion of the long process of the incus. If the incudostapedial joint is intact, it is divided with a joint knife and the incus carefully removed without damaging the stapes superstructure. The neck of the malleus is then divided with malleus nippers and the head of the malleus removed; the handle of malleus can either be removed or left *in situ*. Removal of the handle of malleus can make reconstruction simpler and reduce recurrent cholesteatoma.

5 Cortical mastoidectomy – Using a 5 or 6 mm cutting burr, the cortical bone is removed to make a cavity (Figure 16.2g–h), the superior margin of which is the tegmen tympani, posterior margin the sigmoid sinus and anterior margin the bony wall of the external auditory canal (Figure 16.2i). As bone is removed, air cells will come into view depending on the degree of sclerosis of the mastoid. It is important to find the tegmen and sigmoid sinus and then skeletonize them (leave a thin layer of bone) with a diamond burr. This ensures that optimal access is achieved and that the surgeon does not become lost down a deep dark hole. The bone of the posterior canal is thinned while looking into the cavity and down the EAC. Anterosuperiorly, the dissection continues forward with a smaller cutting burr into the root of the zygomatic process between the tegmen and bone of the superior EAC to provide access to the attic. With progressive bone removal, the mastoid antrum is encountered. With the mastoid antrum open, the bony bulge of the lateral semicircular canal comes into view, as does the lateral process of the incus. Extreme caution is required as drilling on

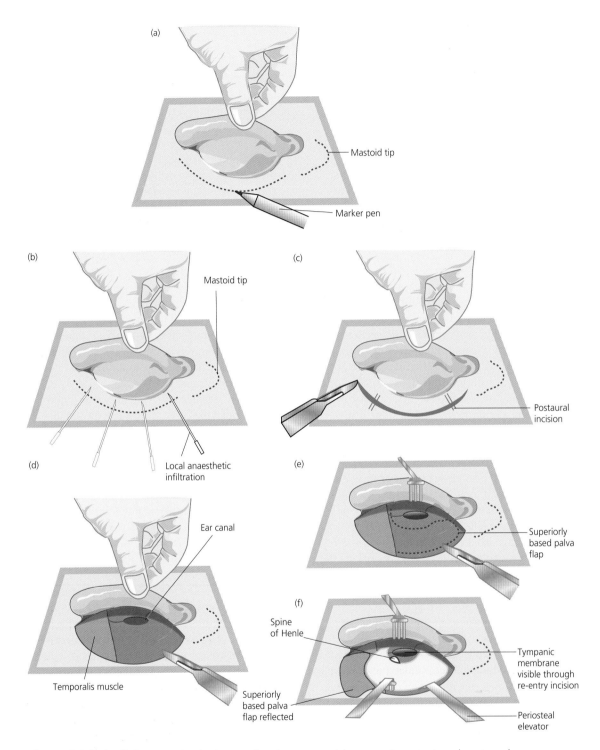

Figure 16.2. (a–f) Steps involved when performing a mastoidectomy via a postaural approach.

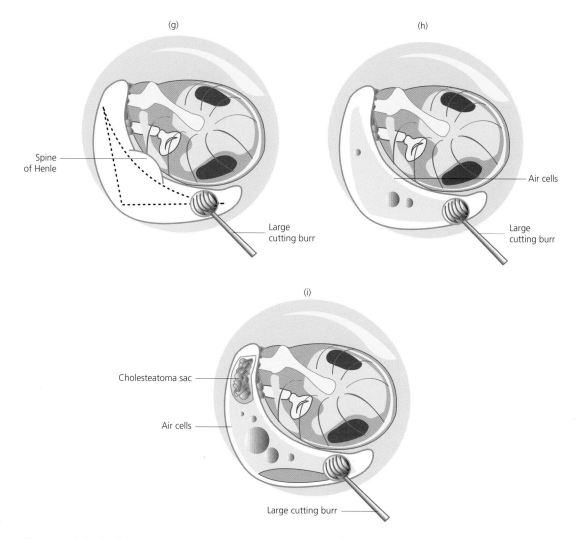

(g)

Spine
of Henle

Large
cutting burr

(h)

Air cells

Large
cutting burr

(i)

Cholesteatoma sac

Air cells

Large cutting burr

Figure 16.2. (g–i) Steps involved when performing a mastoidectomy via a postaural approach.

an intact ossicular chain may result in a sensori-neural hearing loss. The dissection is continued anteriorly until the anterior attic is accessible; this can otherwise be a common site for residual disease. Throughout the procedure, cholestea-toma and granulations may require piecemeal removal in order to maintain visualization. The final cavity should be smooth and disease-free.

6 Posterior tympanotomy – This refers to the removal of the triangle of bone between the facial nerve, chorda tympani and fossa incudis

(Figure 16.1b) and is best performed with a small diamond burr. The first step is to find the mastoid segment of the facial nerve while drill-ing parallel to it with copious irrigation. Once located, it is possible to remove the bone lateral to the nerve in order to encounter the intra-osseous chorda. By removing the bone between the facial nerve and chorda tympani, the facial recess is opened, providing a view of the stapes (if present) and sinus tympani. In addition to the anterior attic, the sinus tympani is a frequent site for residual cholesteatoma; a good posterior tympanotomy provides optimal visualization of this tricky area, which can be supplemented with angled otoscopes.

7 Tympanic membrane reconstruction – A composite cartilage graft (cartilage and perichondrium) is an excellent material for this and has a high resilience to retraction without adversely affecting hearing outcomes (1). Cartilage is harvested from the concha cymba or concha cavum via the postauricular incision. The posterior bony annulus and attic are smoothed off. A tape passed through the canal and brought out through the mastoid cavity can be used to remove residual squames from the bony margin. A paper template is prepared to size the attic and tympanic membrane reconstruction required. This is done prior to harvesting the cartilage to ensure a large enough piece of cartilage is taken. Once harvested, the cartilage is shaped to the template (taking care to place the lateral aspect of the template on the cartilage) leaving a peripheral apron of perichondrium surrounding the cartilage. The cartilage is scored down to perichondrium, twice horizontally and twice vertically. The result is nine separate pieces, resembling a chessboard, that are attached to the perichondrium. This technique removes the natural convexity of conchal cartilage and makes the graft easier to manipulate in the ear. The graft is placed in the middle ear in an underlay fashion with the perichondrium laterally. The perichondrium is placed over the bony meatal wall lateral to the bony annulus, but medial to the annular ligament and tympanomeatal flap to anchor the graft and prevent medialization. The cartilage should extend snugly to the bony annulus but not overlap it.

8 Ossiculoplasty – A partial or total ossicular replacement prosthesis (typically titanium or hydroxyapetite) is positioned to bridge the ossicular gap between the tympanic membrane and stapes head or footplate respectively.

The head of the prosthesis lies against the undersurface of the cartilage checkerboard.

9 Ear packing – The surface of the reconstructed tympanic membrane is gently covered with small pieces of BIPP ribbon gauze. The ossiculopasty is inspected via the posterior tympanotomy to ensure that this remains in an optimal position prior to filling the external auditory canal with additional short strips of BIPP ribbon gauze.

10 Closure – The post-auricular wound is closed in layers with absorbable sutures and a head bandage with mastoid dressing is placed overnight.

Postoperatively, the facial nerve function is documented. A postoperative lower motor neurone palsy is extremely worrying and the operating surgeon must be informed. While the palsy may be due to the local anesthetic, if the nerve fails to recover, surgical exploration by the operating surgeon and a second senior otologist is required. Facial nerve reanastamosis may be attempted.

A Weber test or scratch test is also performed to confirm that there is still hearing in the operated ear. While the majority of mastoidectomy cases require an overnight stay, they may be performed as day case procedures.

The patient is advised to keep their ear dry until after review. Postoperative follow-up is usually two weeks after surgery, at which time the dressings are removed. Postoperative antibiotics are not usually necessary.

REFERENCE

1 Dornhoffer J (2003). Cartilage tympanoplasty: indications, techniques and outcomes in a 1,000 patient series. *Laryngoscope* **113**(11): 1844–56.

17

STAPEDECTOMY

Stapedectomy literally means the surgical removal of the stapes bone. The term has come to refer to the operation in which the stapes superstructure is replaced by an artificial piston attached to the incus (typically) and placed through a fenestration in the stapes footplate (stapedotomy). This procedure is used to correct the conductive hearing loss that arises as a result of otosclerosis (Figure 17.1).

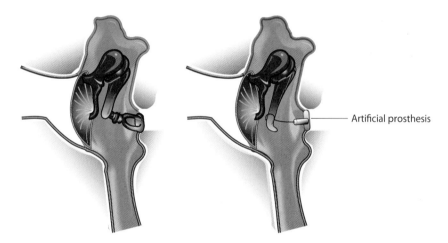

Figure 17.1. Stapedectomy typically involves removal of the stapes crura, fenestration of the footplate and the insertion of an artificial piston.

Otosclerosis affects the bone of the otic capsule, leading to new bone formation around the edge of the oval window and stapes footplate. Eventually, the stapes becomes fixed, resulting in reduced transmission of sound to the cochlea and significant conductive hearing loss.

ASSESSMENT

▌ History

The typical presenting symptom of otosclerosis is hearing loss. Less often there may be associated tinnitus or vertigo. It is commonly (70%) a bilateral condition in patients with a family history of hearing loss. Otosclerosis genes are transmitted in an autosomal-dominant manner. However, due to variable penetrance and expression, it does not affect every generation.

▊ Examination

Tuning fork tests are useful to confirm clinically a conductive hearing loss. It is necessary to document the state of both ears and exclude other causes of conductive hearing loss (e.g., otitis media with effusion or a retraction pocket with ossicular erosion). In active disease, hypervascularity of the promontory may be seen as a pinkish blush through the tympanic membrane. This is known as Schwartze's sign.

▊ Investigations

Pure tone audiometry, including air conduction and appropriately masked bone conduction, is an essential part of the assessment. In early disease, a predominantly low-frequency conductive hearing loss is found. With increased fixation of the stapes,

higher frequencies become affected. There may be a mixed conductive and sensorineural loss if there is additional cochlear otosclerosis. Characteristically, a Carhart's notch is seen where a dip in the bone conduction occurs maximally at 2 kHz due to the loss of the middle ear component of sound conduction at this natural frequency of resonance of the ossicular chain.

Tympanometry demonstrates a normal, type A tympanogram confirming normal middle ear compliance. Stapedial reflexes are typically absent on the affected side.

Speech audiometry can be a useful investigation, particularly in the presence of a mixed hearing loss. Maximum speech discrimination scores (SDS) of less than 70% may be associated with a poorer perceived benefit from surgery.

AIMS OF SURGERY

The principal aims of stapedectomy are to provide the patient with an ear that hears to the best of its ability. The probability of improving the hearing to within 10 dB of the bone conduction is >90%.

ALTERNATIVES TO SURGERY

In addition to discussing surgery, it is important to advise patients of the alternatives available to them. Many patients will elect for observation once the diagnosis has been made. A trial of a hearing aid is a risk-free and effective option that should be encouraged prior to electing for surgery.

Complications

The risks of surgery include:

- Bleeding.
- Infection.
- Chorda tympani injury with taste disturbance.
- Dead ear or hearing loss (approximately 1%).
- Failure to close the air–bone gap within 10 dB (approximately 5%).
- Late failure.
- Tinnitus.
- Vertigo.
- Facial nerve injury (rare).

OPERATION

The side to be operated on should be clearly marked and the risks of the procedure explained. The ear must be dry, with no active infection. A recent (within three months) audiogram should also be present.

Check the availability of any specialist equipment with the scrub team. This includes an adequate selection of the preferred stapedectomy prosthesis and, depending on the technique used, a KTP laser with an appropriately trained operator.

As with other otological procedures, ensure the anaesthetist is aware of the need for intraoperative facial nerve monitoring and relative hypotension to reduce bleeding.

The patient is placed supine, with their head on a head ring, rotated away from the operative ear. A small sandbag is placed beneath the shoulders to extend the neck as this makes it easier to access the posterosuperior region of the tympanic membrane. As with other ontological cases, facial nerve monitoring and strapping the patient to the table can be useful adjuncts.

▌ Stapedectomy

Procedure steps

1 Injection of local anaesthetic – Local anaesthetic (e.g., 2% xylociane with 1:80 000 adrenaline) is used to infiltrate the canal skin in order to thicken the tympanomeatal flap and reduce bleeding. It is common practice in many clinics to perform the entire procedure under local anaesthesia, with a peri-auriclar block.
2 Incision – Typically a permeatal or endaural approach is used.
3 Tympanomeatal flap – A posterior bucket handle incision is made, extending from the 12 o'clock position of the TM to the 6 o'clock position. The meatal incision should not be too close to the annulus as it is often necessary to remove some of the bony annulus. The tympanomeatal flap is raised, providing access to the posterior contents of the mesotymanum and allowing the flap to be hinged along the malleus and out of the way. A view of the long process of incus, incudostapedial joint, stapedius tendon and stapes footplate is required. If access is limited, a House curette is used to remove the bone posterior and superior to the stapes until the desired view is achieved (Figure 17.2a).
4 Check of the ossicular chain – Palpate the ossicular chain with a needle. Confirm that the stapes footplate is fixed and that the malleus and incus are mobile.
5 Division of the incudostapedial joint (ISJ) – The ISJ is divided with a joint knife or fine right-angled hook. The joint can be clearly identified by gently elevating the incus. Division of the joint should be in line with and away from the stapedius tendon (Figure 17.2b).
6 Division of the stapedius tendon – The stapedius tendon is divided with a laser, sharp sickle knife or microscissors.
7 Removal of stapes superstructure – The posterior crus of the stapes is divided with a laser or skeeter drill. The anterior crus is divided by down-fracturing towards the promontory.
8 Fenestration – A small fenestration (stapedotomy) is made in the stapes footplate using a skeeter drill, laser or hand-held trephine. The fenestration typically has a diameter of 0.8 or 0.7 mm to accommodate a 0.6 mm prosthesis (Figure 17.2c).
9 Prosthesis – A stapedectomy prosthesis is placed within the fenestration and secured around the long process of the incus. Small pieces of fat, harvested from the ear lobule, are placed around the prosthesis to prevent leakage of perilymph. A vein graft may be placed over the fenestration to perform the same task (Figure 17.2d).
10 Ear packing – The tympanomeatal flap is replaced and the ear lightly packed with small pieces of BIPP ribbon gauze.

POSTOPERATIVE REVIEW

The facial nerve function is documented and a Weber test is performed to confirm that there is still hearing in the operated ear. The eyes are examined and any nystagmus noted. While some stapedectomy cases require an overnight stay, increasing numbers are being performed as day case procedures.

The patient is given advice to keep their ear dry until after review. Postoperative follow-up is usually two weeks after surgery, at which time the dressings are removed.

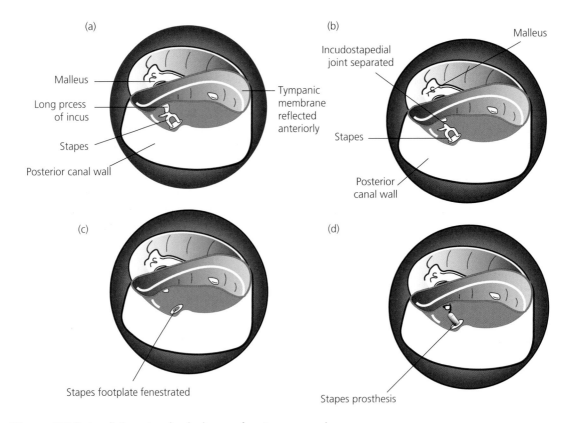

Figure 17.2. (a–d) Steps involved when performing a stapedectomy.

18

BONE-ANCHORED HEARING AID

A bone-anchored hearing aid (BAHA) provides hearing rehabilitation through bone conduction. The BAHA consists of a titanium implant, abutment and a sound processor. The implant is placed surgically behind the ear and forms a solid attachment to bone through osseointegration. The sound processor is removable and facilitates sound conduction through vibrations, which are transmitted via the abutment and implant complex through the skull to reach the cochlea. BAHA offers superior sound quality to a conventional bone conductor hearing aid.

Indications

● Patients unable to wear a conventional hearing aid due to otitis externa, chronically discharging ears, allergy to hearing aid moulds or congenital malformation of the middle or external ear, including canal and pinna atresia.
● Unilateral complete sensorineural hearing loss. Placed behind the deaf ear, the BAHA facilitates the conduction of sound through the skull to the good ear. This prevents the head shadow effect from the deaf side, although in general does not improve directionality.

PREOPERATIVE REVIEW

Ensure that the patient has completed their audiological assessment for BAHA, which includes a trial of a bone conductor worn on a headband. Mark the side on which the BAHA is to be placed.

OPERATIVE PROCEDURE

This is usually performed under general anaesthetic. Ensure that at least two BAHA implants are available prior to starting (one spare). The patient is positioned supine with the head facing 45° away from the surgeon. Shave the post-auricular area, prepare the skin and drape (Figure 18.1a).

Mark the position of the implant 55 mm from the external auditory meatus in the direction shown (Figure 18.1b). Use the dummy sound processor in order to ensure that the eventual position of the processor will not impinge on the ear and the arm of glasses if worn. Draw around the dummy sound processor in order to mark the skin flap, which is most commonly anteriorly based. Local anaesthesia (2% xylocaine, 1:80 000 adrenaline) is instilled (Figure 18.1c).

The skin flap may be raised manually (full thickness) or with a dermatome (split skin). Use a no. 15 scalpel blade to incise the skin alone (Figure 18.1d).

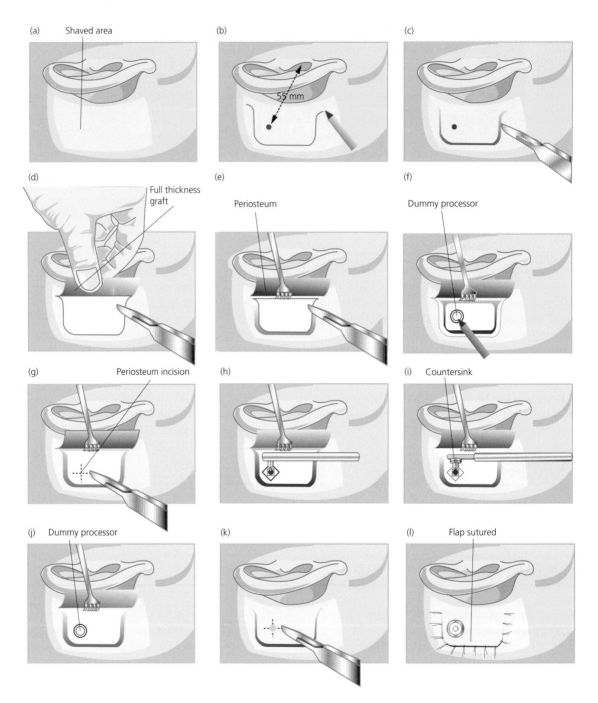

Figure 18.1. (a) Post-auricular shave. (b) Marking implant position. (c) Incision. (d) Raising flap. (e) Excision of subcutaneous fat. (f) Marking abutment site. (g) Periosteal incision. (h) Drilling guide hole. (i) Countersink. (j) Placing abutment. (k) Incision for abutment. (l) Closure.

Carefully raise a full thickness skin flap, ensuring that no fat is left on the flap and the hair follicles are transected (Figure 18.1e).

Excise all subcutaneous fat down to, but preserving, the skull periosteum (Figure 18.1f). Angle the blade at 45° to undermine fat under the skin edges in order to ensure that the implant and hearing aid are not in contact with the skin.

Mark the implant position again using the dummy hearing aid (Figure 18.1f).

Make a cruciate incision in the periosteum and elevate each corner (Figure 18.1g).

Drill the hole for the implant, using the hand-held drill. Ensure that the irrigation is on and drill speed high. Initially, drill a guide hole 3 mm deep perpendicular to the skull. Palpate the base of the hole carefully. If bone remains, redrill the hole to a depth of 4 mm (Figure 18.1h).

One-stage implants are used in the majority of cases, consisting of the implant screw and abutment as one unit (Figure 18.1i). A two-stage technique may be used in children, where the implant alone is initially placed under the skin and an abutment screwed onto this three months later after osseointegration has taken place. Mount the implant onto the drill using a no-touch technique. The implant is a self-tapping screw. Turn the irrigation off and set the torque of the drill to 20 N/m^2. It is essential that this is placed perpendicular to the skull. Insert the implant into the hole and, after the first couple of turns, restart the irrigation. Do not stop the drill until the implant stops turning (Figure 18.1j).

Cut a hole in the overlying skin with a 4 mm dermatological punch and make radial incisions in order to enable the abutment to pass through the skin (Figure 18.1k).

Place the healing cap firmly onto the abutment and suture the skin (Figure 18.1l). Place a non-adherent dressing and foam under the healing cap for one week. A head bandage compression dressing overnight is optional.

POSTOPERATIVE REVIEW AND FOLLOW-UP

Following observation according to the day surgery protocol, the patient can be discharged with analgesia. Initial follow-up is at one week to remove the healing cap and change the dressings. Further dressing changes may be performed by nursing staff. The patient is taught to care for their implant, which requires daily cleaning with a soft toothbrush. The hearing aid is fitted and programmed after three months.

Complications

● Infection.
● Bleeding or haematoma.
● Failure of skin graft.
● Failure of implant.

19
PANENDOSCOPY

Panendoscopy refers to the formal assessment of the upper aero-digestive tract using rigid endoscopes. The term encompasses a number of distinct procedures:

- Examination of the postnasal space (PNS).
- Pharyngoscopy.
- Laryngoscopy.
- Rigid oesophagoscopy.

On occasion, a rigid bronchoscopy may be required to complete a formal assessment of the upper aero-digestive tract.

PREOPERATIVE REVIEW

All imaging must be reviewed. Patients at risk of cervical spine injury should undergo a cervical spine x-ray. Loose teeth or dental crowns require extra precautions to prevent damage. Mouth opening and neck movement are assessed in the awake patient as this will impact on the ease of the procedure.

OPERATIVE PROCEDURE

The light source and carrier are checked to make certain they are functioning correctly. An appropriate range of endoscopes, Hopkins rods and a variety of biopsy forceps must be available.

The procedure is undertaken under general anaesthetic and the patient placed supine on the operating table. Either a pillow or head ring and shoulder roll are used to allow the neck to be slightly flexed and the head extended to achieve the 'sniffing the morning air' position. The endotracheal or nasotracheal tube is secured, the former being secured on the left if the surgeon is right hand-dominant.

The eyes are taped closed and the head draped with the nose and mouth exposed. The body is draped leaving the neck exposed.

In all cases, the neck is inspected for scars and the neck palpated for masses and laryngeal crepitus. The oral cavity, tongue base and tonsils are also palpated. For all procedures, except examination of the PNS, an appropriate mouth guard is placed to protect the upper teeth. If the patient is edentulous a wet swab will suffice.

Biopsies, if required, are taken distal to proximal in order to ensure that bleeding does not obscure the surgeon's view.

20 DIRECT- AND MICRO-LARYNGOSCOPY

Indications

- Laryngeal pathology (e.g., laryngeal carcinoma, laryngeal polyp, cord oedema).
- Investigation of a patient with an unknown primary.
- Investigation of a patient with dysphagia.
- Investigation of an unknown cause for airway symptoms.
- Removal of a foreign body.
- Investigation and management of a patient with a vocal cord palsy.
- Paediatric airway assessment.

OPERATIVE PROCEDURE

The patient is intubated with a micro-laryngeal tube, which is of a standard length but smaller diameter to allow better visualization.

The mouth is held open with the non-dominant hand. The laryngoscope is gently inserted and the tongue followed until the oropharynx is reached, with any secretions suctioned.

The endotracheal tube acts as a guide and can be followed directly to the larynx. Inspect the lingual and laryngeal surfaces of the epiglottis and the remainder to the supraglottis, including the arytenoids. Once the vocal cords, including the anterior commissure, are visible, the laryngoscope handle can be attached and the suspension arm fixed to the handle to support the laryngoscope when micro-laryngoscopy is required. An anterior commisure laryngoscope, which has a narrower cross-sectional profile, may be required to allow assessment of the anterior commisure.

A 0° Hopkins rod is passed through the lumen of the laryngoscope. Careful assessment is made of the supraglottis, glottis and subglottis and appropriate photographs taken. In paediatric patients, a probe is used to assess mobility of the cords and the crico-arytenoid joints. Representative biopsies can be taken from any lesions.

The operating microscope can now be used if the following procedures are undertaken:

- A magnified view of the larynx is required to allow accurate excision of a lesion or vocal cord injection.
- Both hands are required to perform the procedure.
- Laser excision of a laryngeal lesion.

Complications

- Bleeding.
- Infection.
- Damage to teeth, gums, lips and tongue.
- Hoarse voice.
- Sore throat.
- Dysphagia.
- Airway compromise, which may necessitate tracheostomy.

POSTOPERATIVE REVIEW

- If the patient is difficult to intubate and there is a high likelihood that the airway will be unstable on extubation, a tracheostomy should be undertaken.
- If there is any concern that the airway may be compromised, then extubation is performed in theatre and assessment of the airway undertaken prior to transfer to recovery. If there is any concern, re-intubation and tracheostomy may be required.

Patients are advised to rest their voice for at least 48 hours or talk normally with no shouting or whispering.

21
PHARYNGOSCOPY

Indications

- Mass or ulcer of the oropharynx and hypopharynx.
- Investigation of a patient with an unknown primary.
- Dysphagia.
- Identifying a synchronous tumour in a patient with known malignancy of the upper aero-digestive tract.
- Removal of a foreign body.
- Globus sensation, failing to respond to medical therapy or with features suggestive of malignancy on history, examination or imaging.

OPERATIVE PROCEDURE

The non-dominant hand is used to gently open the mouth and the pharyngoscope inserted (Figure 21.1). The tongue will guide the surgeon inferiorly towards the oropharynx. Suction is required at this point, as secretions will obscure the surgical field. The tongue base, valleculae, tonsils, posterior and lateral pharyngeal walls are carefully examined.

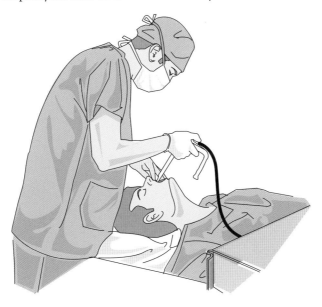

Figure 21.1. Insertion of the pharyngoscope.

The pharyngoscope is passed behind the endo-tracheal or nasotracheal tube in order to visualize the posterior pharyngeal wall, pyriform fossae and post-cricoid region.

It is essential that the surgeon has a clear view at all times. Never attempt to force the pharyngoscope as this risks causing an oesophageal perforation (Figure 21.2). If this leads to mediastinitis, the mortality rate is 50%. At the cricopharyngeal bar, the lumen may come to a blind end and the temptation is to push the scope blindly. Wait patiently for the muscle to relax. Otherwise, the larynx may be gently lifted forward to allow identification of the lumen of the cervical oesophagus. The tip of the scope is advanced gently into the upper oesophagus. A 0° Hopkins rod can be passed through the lumen to take photographs of any abnormality, prior to taking representative biopsies using an appropriate biopsy forceps (Figure 21.3). In patients with an unknown primary malignancy, biopsies of the tongue base and tonsils are usually taken if no obvious primary can be identified.

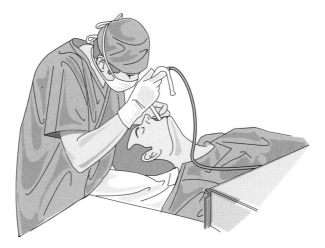

Figure 21.2. At the cripharyngeus, the scope is gently advanced in order to avoid tearing.

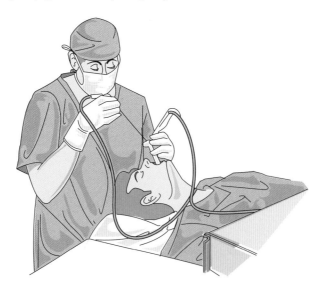

Figure 21.3. Suction is often required once the pharyngoscope is within the cervical oesophagus. Biopsy forceps are required if a biopsy is to be taken.

At the end of the procedure, ensure haemostasis and remove the teeth guard, checking for any dental trauma, which must be documented in the operation note.

POSTOPERATIVE REVIEW

If there is any concern of trauma to the upper oesophagus, a nasogastric tube should be passed under direct vision during the procedure and the patient kept nil by mouth. A contrast swallow allows visualization of a potential perforation. If the suspicion of perforation is low, the patient is observed closely for pain radiating to the back, pyrexia, tachycardia or tachypnoea. If these do not occur, the patient can commence sips of sterile water, gradually building up to free fluids and a soft diet prior to discharge home.

Complications

- Bleeding.
- Infection.
- Damage to teeth, gums, lips or tongue.
- Sore throat.
- Dysphagia.
- Hoarse voice.
- Damage to pharyngeal mucosa, including perforation.

22 RIGID OESOPHAGOSCOPY

Rigid oesophagoscopy is performed in a similar manner to pharyngoscopy. Rigid oesophagoscopes are typically available 25 cm or 40 cm in length, which can reach the gastro-oesophageal junction. It is important to ensure that suction and biopsy forceps of an appropriate length are available.

Indications

● Similar to that for rigid pharyngoscopy.

OPERATIVE PROCEDURE

The procedure is similar to that for rigid pharyngoscopy. The oesophagoscope is manoeuvred into the post-cricoid region. The tip of the oesophagoscope is gently lifted to allow identification of the lumen of the oesophagus and for the scope to be gently passed. Never force the scope, especially if the lumen is not visible.

If an abnormality is identified, use the etched marks on the oesophagoscope to estimate the distance from the incisors and document this in the operation note. Representative biopsies are taken. Carefully assess the mucosa as the oesophagoscope is removed and, if there is any suspicion of a mucosal tear or perforation, a nasogastric tube is passed under direct vision. Complete the procedure by removing the mouth guard and checking the teeth.

POSTOPERATIVE REVIEW

Where there is no suspicion of trauma to the oesophagus, patients can eat and drink normally. Otherwise, manage the patient as recommended for perforations after pharyngoscopy.

If a patient becomes pyrexic, tachycardic, tachypnoeic or has increasing retrosternal pain radiating through to their back or dysphagia, always assume they have suffered an oesophageal tear. These patients must be kept nil by mouth. They require IV antibiotics (e.g., cefuroxime and metronidazole) and a nasogastric tube will need to be passed by the radiologists. Obtain an urgent chest x-ray to exclude a pneumomediastinum indicative of a tear, and inform a senior member of the team.

Complications

● As for rigid pharyngoscopy, risk of mucosal tear and perforation. Patients should be made aware of the risk of requiring a nasogastric tube and close monitoring in hospital for a few days if a perforation is suspected.

23

EXAMINATION OF THE POSTNASAL SPACE

Indications

- Mass or ulcer of the nasopharynx.
- Investigation of patient with an unknown primary.
- Persistent unilateral middle ear effusion in an adult.
- Unexplained epistaxis.

OPERATIVE PROCEDURE

This procedure is usually undertaken last if it is part of a panendoscopy, as any bleeding from the nasopharynx due to instrumentation can track into and obscure the view of the rest of the upper aero-digestive tract.

The patient is placed supine on the operating table and the head supported with a head ring. A decongestant or topical anaesthetic with adrenaline is applied to the nose, usually in the anaesthetic room.

A 0° Hopkins rod with an appropriate light source is passed into the nasal cavity, and the nasopharynx is carefully examined. The fossa of Rosenmüller in particular must be assessed as this may harbour a malignancy. Biopsies are taken, if indicated, with straight Blakesley-Wilde forceps. Adrenaline-soaked neuropatties or diathermy can be applied if required for haemostasis.

Complications

- Bleeding/epistaxis.
- Infection.
- Otitis media with effusion secondary to inadvertent damage to the Eustachian tube orifice.

24 RIGID BRONCHOSCOPY

Indications

- Removal of foreign body from the trachea or main bronchi.
- Assessment of a tracheal lesion.

In many cases the proximal trachea can be assessed, as described in Chapter 23, with a laryngoscope and 0° Hopkins rod.

OPERATIVE PROCEDURE

Bronchoscopes are available in a number of sizes. Selection of an appropriately sized bronchoscope is essential for paediatric patients. Before the patient is anaesthetized, ensure that the bronchoscope is assembled correctly and that the anaesthetic connectors are compatible. Confirm that the light source is working and that the camera has been attached. Appropriate optical forceps must be available if foreign body removal is required.

Safe bronchoscopy requires good teamwork and communication between the surgeon and the anaesthetist. When the patient is well oxygenated and the anaesthetist feels it is appropriate, the endotracheal tube or laryngeal mask is withdrawn and a mouth guard placed over the upper teeth. The anaesthetic laryngoscope is held in the non-dominant hand and used to visualize the larynx. The bronchoscope is held in the dominant hand and advanced until the larynx is reached. The bronchoscope is rotated through 90° to facilitate passage through the glottic opening

(which minimizes the risk of damage to the vocal cord from the tip of the bronchoscope).

Once the bronchoscope is in the proximal trachea, the anaesthetic circuit is connected and the bronchoscope is advanced towards the carina. By gently turning the head to the left, the bronchoscope can be advanced into the right main bronchus, and vice versa. Secretions can be removed using narrow suction tubing, which can be advanced by an assistant or scrub nurse.

If a foreign body is visualized, it is vital that a small volume of 1:10 000 adrenaline is instilled via the suction tubing to reduce mucosal oedema and allow vasoconstriction. This improves access and minimizes the risk of bleeding, which can make removal of the foreign body very challenging. Appropriate optical forceps are then used to remove the foreign body. The bronchoscope is reinserted to ensure that there are no more foreign bodies and to assess for mucosal damage.

POSTOPERATIVE REVIEW

The patient is recovered in theatre to ensure that there are no breathing difficulties. If there has been mucosal damage, then a chest x-ray (CXR) is performed to exclude a pneumothorax.

Complications

These are similar to those for laryngoscopy. Others include:

- Damage to the vocal cords by the bronchoscope.
- Laryngospasm.
- Breathing difficulties due to airway oedema.
- Pneumothorax due to damage to of the mucosa of the trachea or main bronchi.

25 SUBMANDIBULAR GLAND EXCISION

This is a common surgical procedure performed by both ENT surgeons and oral and maxillofacial surgeons for benign and malignant disease.

Indications

- Recurrent submandibular gland sialadenitis.
- Obstructive sialolithiasis.
- Benign tumours of the gland. If there is any suspicion of malignancy, then a level I neck dissection is more appropriate than simple excision of the gland.
- Following open trauma to the gland, exploration and removal may be necessary to avoid salivary fistula formation.
- Drooling.

PREOPERATIVE REVIEW

Mark the operative side and check the function of the marginal mandibular, lingual and hypoglossal nerves

Complications

- Bleeding.
- Infection.
- Marginal mandibular nerve damage: transient 5–30% (1–3); permanent <1% (1).
- Lingual nerve damage – 2–3% (1, 2, 3).
- Hypoglossal nerve damage.
- Salivary fistula.
- Scar.
- Recurrence (if surgery is for a tumour).
- Retained stone in stump of Wharton's duct.

OPERATIVE PROCEDURE

Once intubated and transferred to the operating table, position the patient supine on a head ring and shoulder roll with a slight head-up tilt. The head is turned to the contralateral side. The skin is appropriately prepared and draped to expose the corner of the mouth, the angle and lower border of the jaw to the superior border of the clavicle to the midline.

Mark the lower border of the mandible and the site of the skin incision, which lies two finger breadths below the lower border of the mandible, in order to avoid the marginal mandibular nerve (Figure 25.1a). The incision, ideally in a skin crease, runs forward from the anterior edge of the sternocleidomastoid muscle and is approximately 5–7 cm in length (Figure 25.1b).

Make an incision through the skin, subcutaneous tissue and platysma. The marginal mandibular nerve can be damaged in the early stages of the procedure.

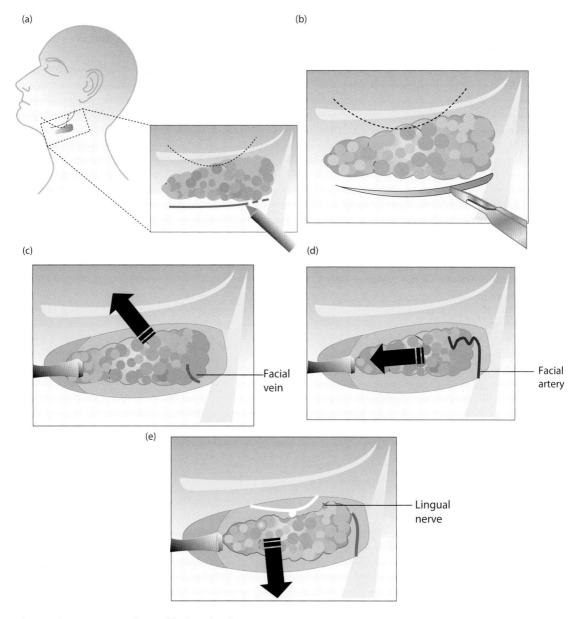

(a)

(b)

(c)

Facial vein

(d)

Facial artery

(e)

Lingual nerve

Figure 25.1. (a–e) Submandibular gland excision.

The nerve does not have to be formerly identified, but knowledge of the relevant clinical anatomy is important as the nerve lies deep to platysma but superficial to the gland and the facial vein.

Stay close to the under-surface of platysma and carefully observe for the nerve when elevating sub-platysmal flaps. The superficial layer of the deep

cervical fascia is incised inferior to the lower border of the gland and elevated in an inferior to superior direction. The facial vein is ligated and divided close to the inferior border of the gland and elevated superiorly away from the gland (Figure 25.1c).

Once the gland is exposed the facial artery is identified, ligated and divided. The gland is retracted and dissected free of the underlying digastric muscle. The posterior border of the mylohyoid muscle is identified and the muscle is retracted anteriorly to allow dissection of the deep aspect of the gland.

The gland is retracted posteroinferiorly and as dissection proceeds, Wharton's duct is exposed, which tents and exposes the lingual nerve and its ganglion (Figure 25.1d). The lingual nerve is dissected off the duct, paying careful attention to haemostasis, especially in the small plexus near the ganglion. The duct is followed and ligated as distally as possible to complete the excision. Occasionally, the facial artery will need to be ligated again as it courses over the mandible. The hypoglossal nerve is identified during dissection of the deep aspect of the gland (Figure 25.1e).

A drain may be inserted and the wound is closed in layers.

POSTOPERATIVE REVIEW

Examine the patient for nerve injury and haematoma. The drain can usually be removed in the morning and the patient discharged home with routine wound care advice.

Non-absorbable skin sutures are removed after seven days.

REFERENCES

1 Preuss SF, Klussmann JP, Wittekindt C, *et al* (2007). Submandibular gland excision: 15 years of experience. *J Oral Maxillofac Surg* **65**(5): 953–7.
2 Chua DY, Ko C, Lu KS (2010). Submandibular mass excision in an Asian population: a 10-year review. *Ann Acad Med Singapore* **39**(1): 33–7.
3 Ichimura K, Nibu K, Tanaka T (1997). Nerve paralysis after surgery in the submandibular triangle: review of University of Tokyo Hospital experience. *Head Neck* **19**(1): 48–53.

26
HEMI- AND TOTAL THYROIDECTOMY

Indications

- Thyroid nodule or goitre.
  - Suspicious (hemi-thyroidectomy) or confirmed (total thyroidectomy) malignancy.
  - Compressive symptoms.
  - Cosmesis.
- Thyrotoxicosis – A total thyroidectomy is usually undertaken.

Complications

- Bleeding.
- Infection.
- Scar.
- Hoarseness due to recurrent laryngeal nerve injury.
- Loss of the upper vocal range due to damage to superior laryngeal nerve injury, which is especially important in singers.
- Breathing difficulties and rarely tracheostomy if bilateral vocal cord palsy after total thyroidectomy.
- Hypocalcaemia.

PREOPERATIVE REVIEW

It is essential that all patients undergo a vocal cord check preoperatively to assess cord movement. Review thyroid function tests and fine needle aspiration cytology (FNAC) results. Thyrotoxic patients are managed jointly with the endocrinologists in order to render them euthyroid to minimize the risk of an intraoperative thyroid storm.

Ensure the correct side is marked in a hemi-thyroidectomy.

OPERATIVE PROCEDURE

The patient is placed supine on the operating table with a shoulder roll and head ring. The skin is prepared and draped.

A horizontal skin crease collar incision is made approximately 1–2 finger breadths above the sternal notch. Marking the incision prior to anaesthesia helps identify an appropriate skin crease.

The incision passes through skin, subcutaneous tissue and platysma (Figure 26.1). Sub-platysmal flaps are elevated as far as the superior thyroid notch superiorly and the supra-sternal notch inferiorly. The anterior jugular veins lie within the sub-platysmal plane and may require ligation and division. A Joll's retractor or sutures are used to retract the flaps out of the operative field.

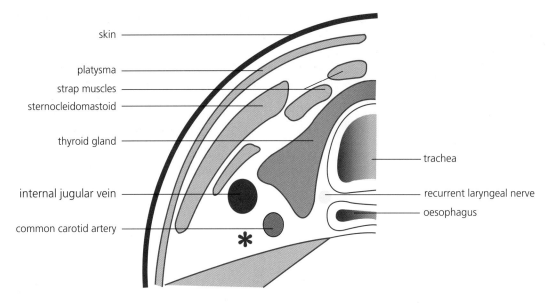

skin

platysma

strap muscles

sternocleidomastoid

thyroid gland

internal jugular vein

common carotid artery

trachea

recurrent laryngeal nerve

oesophagus

*

Figure 26.1. Axial section through the neck at the level of the thyroid isthmus. The vagus nerve is represented by the asterisk.

The investing layer of deep fascia is incised and the strap muscles (sternothyroid and sternohyoid) lying in the midline will come into view. The strap muscles are separated in the midline. Sternothyroid may occasionally need to be divided for large goitres. This is performed as high as possible to preserve innervation from ansa hypoglossi.

The strap muscles are retracted laterally and the underlying gland dissected free using a combination of sharp and blunt dissection. The gland is freed in the para-carotid tunnel and the straps and carotid retracted laterally.

The superior pole is dissected from an inferior to superior direction. The superior vascular pedicle is isolated, ligated and divided close to the gland to minimize damage to the superior laryngeal nerve. This allows the superior pole to be freed from its fascial attachments.

The thyroid gland is retracted medially, which also rotates the larynx, exposing the tracheo-oesophageal groove. The middle thyroid vein is identified and divided. The recurrent laryngeal nerve (RLN) lies in the tracheo-oesophageal groove and has a variable course, but always enters the larynx at the

cricothyroid joint. Safe identification of the RLN can be made in several ways including:

● The RLN runs within Beahr's triangle, which is formed by the common carotid, inferior thyroid artery and the recurrent laryngeal nerve. The RLN runs within Lore's triangle, which is formed by the trachea, the carotid sheath and the under-surface of the inferior lobe of the thyroid.
● The RLN is related to the inferior thyroid artery, which is identified laterally at the external carotid and followed medially. The nerve is usually deep to the artery, but can be superficial or between its branches.
● Identify the RLN superiorly just before it enters the larynx caudal to the inferior pharyngeal constrictor.

Once the nerve has been identified, it is followed until it enters the larynx and the thyroid is carefully dissected free. It is vital that the parathyroid glands are identified and dissected free from the thyroid with their blood supply. Divide the inferior thyroid artery close to the thyroid gland to help achieve this.

The thyroid gland remains attached to the trachea by Berry's ligament, a dense fascial condensation.

This is usually vascular and the gland is freed to the midline using bipolar and sharp dissection. If a hemi-thyroidectomy is being performed, the isthmus is divided and over-sewn or transfixed. If a total thyroidectomy is being performed, then the other lobe is excised in a similar fashion.

Haemostasis is achieved with the careful use of bipolar diathermy and great care taken around the nerve. A drain is optional if a hemi-thyroidectomy is undertaken but is usually required after total thyroidectomy.

The strap muscles are closed in the midline using an absorbable suture, with a gap left inferiorly to allow blood to escape from around the trachea and minimize the risk of airway obstruction from a haematoma. The wound is closed in layers, with an absorbable suture for platysma and a subcuticular suture or staples to skin.

POSTOPERATIVE REVIEW

A patient undergoing a total thyroidectomy or with a known vocal cord palsy is extubated in theatre and the patient's airway assessed prior to transfer to recovery.

Voice and cough should be assessed postoperatively. A bovine cough or weak and breathy voice indicates a RLN injury, which should be confirmed by naso-endoscopy. Clip removers or scissors must always be at the patient's bedside to enable immediate evacuation of a haematoma should this occur (this may compromise the airway).

If a completion hemi-thyroidectomy or total thyroidectomy has been undertaken, postoperative calcium levels may be checked after 4–6 hours and again the following morning. If the calcium is low, then the local protocol is followed in conjunction with the endocrinology team. Calcium may be replaced orally or, if very low, intravenously, with the addition of 1-α calcidol as required. The patient is also commenced on thyroid replacement with either levothyroxine (T_4) or, where radio-active iodine is to be administered within the following six weeks, liothyronine (T_3). If a drain has been inserted, it is left in place overnight and removed when less than 20 mL has drained in a 24-hour period. The patient is discharged home once the drain has been removed and, if applicable, when the calcium is normal.

Vocal cord movement is assessed at outpatient follow-up.

27

SUPERFICIAL PAROTIDECTOMY

The plane of the facial nerve divides the parotid gland anatomically into superficial deep lobes, although they are functionally the same gland. The majority of parotid tumours occur in the superficial lobe. Superficial parotidectomy is excision of the parotid gland superficial to the facial nerve.

Indications

- Benign or malignant tumour of the parotid gland (most common).
- Chronic sialadenitis (rare).
- Sialolithiasis (rare).

Complications

- Bleeding.
- Infection.
- Facial weakness.
- Numbness of the ear lobe secondary to damage to the greater auricular nerve. This is to be expected in the majority of patients.
- Frey's syndrome. The cut parasympathetic nerve fibres re-innervate the sympathetic channels to supply the sweat glands in the cheek. Gustatory sweating occurs, which is sweating of the face on the side of surgery in anticipation of eating.
- Recurrence of tumour.
- Scar.
- Salivary fistula.

PREOPERATIVE REVIEW

Always check and document facial nerve function preoperatively (Figure 27.1). Review imaging and FNAC results and ensure that any preoperative blood test results are available.

OPERATIVE PROCEDURE

Once the patient has been intubated and transferred to the operating table a head ring is placed under the head, a sandbag under the shoulder, and the head turned to the opposite side.

Facial nerve monitoring is used by most surgeons. Be familiar with the facial nerve monitor used in the unit by practicing placement of the electrodes, connection to the monitor and checking correct function.

A cotton wool ball may be placed in the EAC and the patient prepared with aqueous iodine or chlorhexidine and draped to ensure that the majority of the face is exposed.

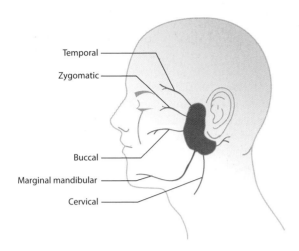

Figure 27.1. External branches of the facial nerve.

The most common incision used is the 'lazy S' incision (Figure 27.2), although a face lift incision is becoming more popular. Infiltration with adrenaline alone, or local anaesthetic and adrenaline, may be used to provide some haemostasis.

Once the incision has been made, an anterior skin flap is raised between the parotid gland capsule and superficial fat layer. The platysma can be used to identify the correct plane inferiorly. The flap over the parotid gland can be raised using a blade or scissors. Good retraction helps identify the plane to prevent a breach through the skin, gland or tumour capsule. As the anterior border of the parotid gland is reached care must be taken to prevent damage to the branches of the facial nerve as they emerge from the gland. The flap is retracted anteriorly with sutures.

The sternocleidomastoid muscle is identified and its anterior border dissected free. The greater auricular nerve will be encountered. It is sometimes possible to preserve a posterior branch that supplies sensation to the ear lobe. The posterior belly of the digastric muscle is exposed and traced back to its insertion into the mastoid. The perichondrium of the tragus is identified and the tragus exposed to its deep extent to reveal the tragal pointer. Another suture retracts the ear lobule posteriorly. The parotid gland between the tragus and posterior belly of the digastric is carefully dissected to ensure wide exposure (Figure 27.3).

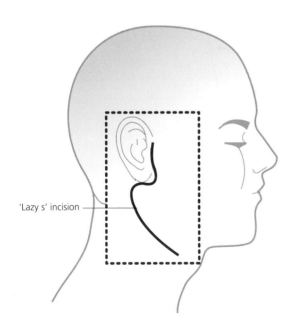

Figure 27.2. Incision landmarks for a parotidectomy.

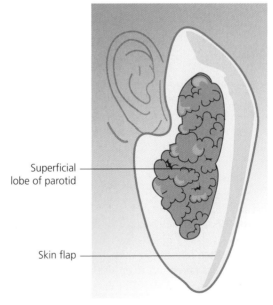

Figure 27.3. Superficial exposure of the parotid gland.

There are several ways to find the facial nerve. A combination of the first three landmarks is usually adequate to ensure safe dissection in the majority of cases:

1 Finding the nerve as it bisects the tympanomastoid groove. This is the most constant landmark.
2 Using the tragal pointer, the nerve lies approximately 1 cm deep and 1 cm inferior to the tragal pointer.
3 The nerve lies just deep and superior to the posterior belly of digastric near its attachment to the mastoid.
4 Where a large tumour lies directly over the proximal aspect of the facial nerve, find a distal branch, such as the marginal mandibular, and follow the nerve in a retrograde manner.
5 Where the above measures fail, drill into the mastoid portion of the temporal bone to identify the descending portion of the facial nerve and follow it out of the stylomastoid foramen.

Careful dissection on a broad front with precise use of bipolar diathermy to ensure complete haemostasis will allow identification of the facial nerve trunk (Figure 27.4), which can be confirmed by use of a nerve stimulator. The main trunk typically divides into upper and lower divisions, which divide in a variety of combinations into the five terminal branches. There is often some cross-communication between the branches. Each branch of the facial nerve is followed using a small, curved clip to dissect the gland from the nerve. The gland may then be cut superficial to the nerve under direct vision using either a no. 12 scalpel or scissors. Bipolar diathermy must be used precisely to prevent thermal damage to branches of the facial nerve. Parotid

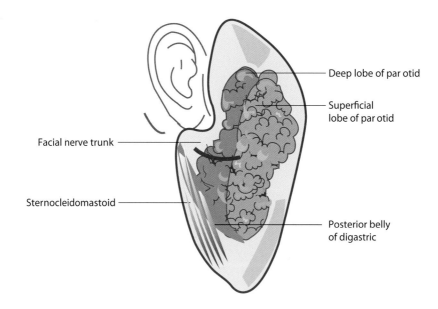

Figure 27.4. Identification of the facial nerve trunk.

tumours often lie directly over branches of the nerve. Care is taken not to enter the tumour, as this risks recurrence at a later date.

The parotid gland is carefully dissected free of the facial nerve, preserving all branches. Very

rarely, when no other option is available, one or more branches of the facial nerve may have to be sacrificed. A drain is usually required and an absorbable suture used to close platysma, with the skin closed with a non-absorbable monofilament suture or staples.

POSTOPERATIVE REVIEW

Always check and document facial nerve function postoperatively and exclude a haematoma. The drain will usually be left in place at least overnight. The patient can be discharged home once the drain has been removed.

Sutures or skin staples are usually removed at 5–7 days with a follow-up arranged to review histology in the clinic.

28 TRACHEOSTOMY

A tracheostomy is a conduit from the skin of the neck to the trachea. It is classically performed in an open surgical fashion, however, more recently percutaneous techniques have been developed and are frequently used. The formation of an open surgical tracheostomy may be required in the emergency or elective setting.

Indications

- Real or anticipated airway obstruction.
- Prolonged ventilation.
- Pulmonary toilet.

METHODS

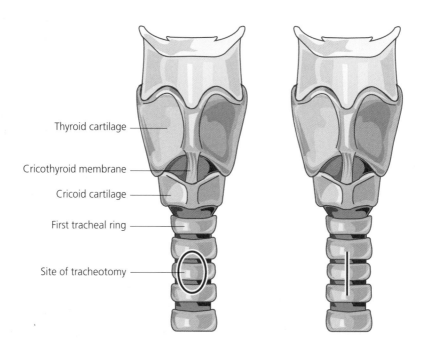

Thyroid cartilage

Cricothyroid membrane

Cricoid cartilage

First tracheal ring

Site of tracheotomy

- Cricothyroidotomy – This may be required in the emergency setting when access to the airway is required. The gap between the thyroid and cricoid cartilages (cricothyroid membrane) is palpated. A horizontal stab incision facilitates the insertion of a mini-tracheostomy.
- Percutaneus tracheostomy – This technique has gained popularity with intensive therapy unit (ITU) interventionists. It is performed using a Seldinger technique, where a guide wire is inserted through a trans-tracheal needle, which has been placed in the midline through the skin into the trachea. A series of dilators are gradually 'railroaded' over this to widen the tract. Finally, the tracheostomy tube can be inserted.

This is often performed with the benefit of a flexible bronchoscope through the larynx from above to ensure correct positioning in the trachea.
- Trans-tracheal needle – Wide-bore needles are available which can be inserted and then connected to a jet ventilation system to maintain an airway. This is a temporary measure to allow oxygenation while a secure airway is inserted. Since it does not allow for expiration, the upper airway should be clear enough to allow for gases to be expired.
- Surgical tracheostomy – This will be considered in greater detail below.

FORMATION OF A SURGICAL TRACHEOSTOMY

A tracheostomy is usually performed under general anaesthesia, although the use of local anaesthesia may be necessary where the airway is too narrow to allow intubation. The skin is infiltrated with local anaesthetic and the tracheal mucosa injected just before an incision is made into the trachea.

The procedure requires the following steps:

1 Patient position – The patient is positioned supine with the head in the midline. A sandbag is placed under the shoulders and a head ring is used to support the head. This extends the neck allowing the laryngeal skeleton and trachea to be readily palpated. It is always prudent to check the tracheostomy tube cuff at this point. A single tube may be chosen at the start of the procedure, but a variety of sizes should be available.
2 Skin incision – A skin incision is made halfway between the cricoid and the suprasternal notch and extended through platysma (Figure 28.1). The anterior jugular veins and midline strap muscles will now come in to view (Figure 28.2).
3 Identification of the thyroid gland and trachea – The strap muscles are separated in the midline and retracted, bringing the trachea and thyroid isthmus into view (Figure 28.3).
4 Division of the thyroid gland – The thyroid gland is clamped through the isthmus, divided in the midline and a transfixion suture used to prevent bleeding. With the thyroid isthmus divided, the trachea will be better exposed.
5 A window into the trachea is fashioned – Inform the anaesthetist before entering the trachea. There are a number of methods of entering the trachea. In children, a vertical slit is made in the midline and stay sutures placed either side of the incision. These sutures are taped to the child's chest and used to hold open the hole if the tracheostomy tube displaces or when the tracheostomy tube is first changed at seven days. In adults, a window is cut just large enough to admit the tracheostomy tube. In both cases the cricoid cartilage must not be injured. For this reason, the window or incision is made through the 2nd, 3rd or 4th tracheal rings (Figure 28.4).
6 A tracheostomy tube is inserted – Ask the anaesthetist to deflate the cuff and withdraw the endotracheal tube until the tip is just above the window. The tracheostomy tube may be inserted, the cuff inflated and the tube sutured into place and appropriate dressings applied.

If an emergency tracheostomy is required, it is essential to gain access and maintain the airway as quickly as possible. In these cases, a vertical midline incision is made to avoid all vascular structures except the thyroid, which must be dealt with rapidly in the emergency scenario.

(a)

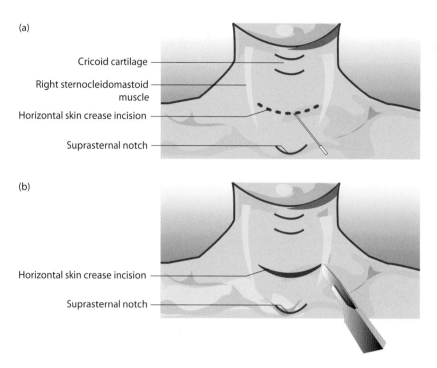

Cricoid cartilage

Right sternocleidomastoid muscle

Horizontal skin crease incision

Suprasternal notch

(b)

Horizontal skin crease incision

Suprasternal notch

Figure 28.1. Tracheostomy incision.

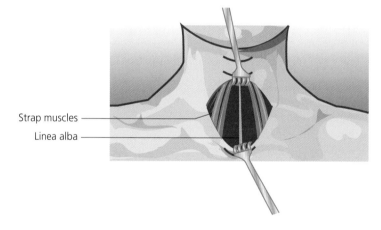

Strap muscles

Linea alba

Figure 28.2. Identification of thyroid isthmus.

Complications

These may classified as immediate, early and late.

Immediate (within 24 hours of procedure)
Haemorrhage – thyroid vessels; jugular veins.
Pneumothorax.
Air embolism.

Cardiac arrest
Local damage to thyroid cartilage, cricoid cartilage, recurrent laryngeal nerve(s).
Dislodgement or displacement of the tube.

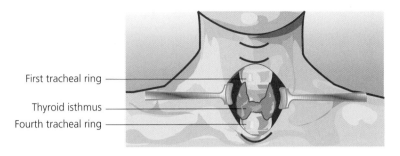

First tracheal ring

Thyroid isthmus

Fourth tracheal ring

Figure 28.3. Division of thyroid isthmus.

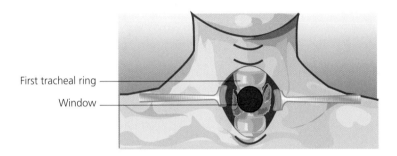

First tracheal ring

Window

Figure 28.4. Tracheal window.

Early (24 hours–7 days)
Dislodgement or displacement of tube.
Surgical emphysema of neck.
Crusting.
Infection.
Tracheal necrosis.
Tracheo-arterial fistula.

Tracheo-oesophageal fistula.
Dysphagia.

Late (after seven days)
Tracheal stenosis.
Difficulty with decannulation.
Tracheo-cutaneous fistula.

TRACHEOSTOMY TUBE CARE AND SPEAKING VALVES

Tracheostomy tube care is often left to tracheostomy nurse specialists or members of the nursing staff. It is, however, essential that junior doctors are able to care for patients with tracheostomy tubes in place and are aware of the potential complications of having a tracheostomy. It is often the case that out-of-hours emergencies and advice will be directed towards the junior on-call surgeon.

All patients should have a spare tracheostomy tube of the same size and one smaller, a tracheal dilator, a 10 mL syringe, a suction unit and catheters, gloves, Spencer-Wells forceps and lubrication for the tubes at their bedside.

▌ Tracheostomy tubes

● Cuffed.
● Uncuffed.
● Fenestrated.
● With or without an inner cannula.
● Adjustable flange.

A tracheostomy tube can be directly attached to an anaesthetic circuit provided that there is a 15 mm connector at the proximal end. Some tubes have this segment on the inner tube, so this should always be available.

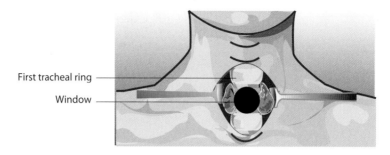

First tracheal ring

Window

Figure 28.5. A cuffed tracheostomy tube.

Cuffed tubes (Figure 28.5)

Advantages:

- A cuff is required for:
  - Ventilation, continuous positive airway pressure.
  - Patients who aspirate as they cannot protect their airway.

Patients with normal swallowing reflexes may find their swallowing impaired as a result of pressure exerted on their oesophagus and the impedance of laryngeal elevation by an inflated cuff.

Disadvantages:

- If the tube lumen becomes blocked, the patient's airway is compromised leading to respiratory arrest as there is no capacity to breathe around the tube, unless the cuff is deflated.
- The cuff can damage the tracheal mucosa, leading to ulceration and possible stenosis. Rarely, this may also cause arterial erosion.
- Children younger than 10 years have a narrow trachea, and unlike in the adult, the larynx is conical, with the cricoid cartilage forming the narrowest segment. Tracheostomy tubes used in children are uncuffed.

$$Pressure = Force/Area$$

High-pressure, low-volume soft cuffs reduce the incidence of pressure-induced complications, but it is still important not to over inflate the cuff.

The cuff should be deflated as soon as possible to allow for the insertion of a speaking tube or decannulation cap.

Uncuffed tubes

These are often found in patients returning from ITU after a prolonged stay as they allow suction and physiotherapy. The tube is easy to replace and suitable for long-term use. Patients can speak around it. They are not suitable for patients who aspirate or who need ventilation.

Fenestrated tubes

The fenestration directs airflow through the patient's vocal cords, oropharynx and nasopharynx. It helps some patients to resume breathing normally and can be used to wean them off their tracheostomy tube. Remember that a fenestrated inner tube is also required.

Tube with adjustable flange (Figure 28.6)

This is designed for patients with deep-set tracheas and fat necks.

The flange can be adjusted to fit the depth of tissue between incision and trachea.

▊ Cleaning inner tubes

Most recommend water or warm salty water only. Avoid alcohol, bleach and glutaldehyde. Flush the tube and do not soak it as this increases the risk of bacterial proliferation.

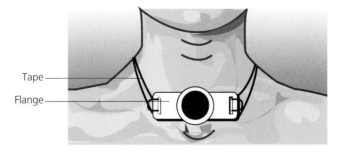

Tape

Flange

Figure 28.6. Tracheostomy tube *in situ*.

Humidification

- Nebulizers 5 mL, 0.9% N/saline in mask over stoma.
- Heat moisture exchangers fit onto the tracheostomy tube.
- Foam filter protectors such as the Buchanon laryngectomy protector.

▊ Tracheostomy dressings

The objective is to keep the trachea, stoma and adjacent skin clean and dry, and minimize skin irritation and infection. Wet skin results in maceration and excoriation. Hydrophilic polyurethane foam dressings absorb moisture away from the skin.

If a tracheostomy site shows signs of granulation, this can be treated with silver nitrate cautery, although care should be taken not to damage surrounding normal skin.

▊ Changing a tracheostomy tube

Most surgeons recommend the first tube change to be performed at one week. The first change should be performed by an experienced practitioner or ideally by the surgeon.

If a difficult tube change is anticipated, use an exchange device (guide wire or a bougie) and consider changing the tube in the operating theatre.

The steps involved are as follows:

1 Explain to the patient what you plan to do. Ensure that a good light source, preferably a headlight, is available.
2 Extend the patient's neck using pillows so the head is supported and hyper-oxygenate them if required.
3 Check the integrity of the cuff if used. Lubricate it sparingly.
4 Remove all old dressings and clean around the stoma site.
5 Remove intraoral secretions with suction, deflate the cuff and suction through the old tube. Some secretions trapped around the cuff will now fall into the trachea inducing coughing.
6 Allow the patient to recover and remove the old tube.
7 Insert a new tube, inflate the cuff if indicated and insert the inner cannula.
8 Check chest movement, insert a clean dressing and apply the tapes before checking cuff pressure.
9 If you are uncertain of the position of the tube, a flexible endoscope can be passed into the trachea through the tube lumen.
10 Connect to any humidification devices.

GENERATING A VOICE

- Cuff deflation.
- Fenestrated tracheostomy tube (and inner tube).
- Smaller tracheostomy tube.
- Intermittent finger occlusion.
- One-way speaking valves.

All of the above allow air to escape around or through the tube into the larynx and the oro-pharynx. One-way speaking valves allow air to be inspired but not exhaled through the tube.

Do not put a one-way speaking valve on a patient with a cuffed fenestrated tube unless their inner tube is also fenestrated. If you do, they will struggle.

It can take time for a patient to get used to a speaking valve, and they need to be encouraged to breathe in through their tracheostomy and out through their mouth. Patients need to be monitored for signs of respiratory distress in the early stages of using a one-way speaking valve.

Contraindictions

- End-stage pulmonary disease.
- Excessive secretions.
- Unstable medical.
- Anarthria.
- Ventilatory status unstable.
- Airway obstruction.
- Severe anxiety or cognitive dysfunction.
- Severe tracheal or laryngeal stenosis.
- Inability to tolerate cuff deflation.

29
VOICE

Voice is the method by which humans predominantly communicate. However, speech also allows us to add emotion and expression to what we communicate. Changes in our voice, therefore, can alter the way we communicate or express ourselves.

The production of voice, however, is not purely based around the larynx as it is essential to have the 'ballast' from the lungs to produce the vibration created at the laryngeal level. This vibratory source creates a sound that is shaped and moulded by the articulators and resonators in the upper aerodigestive tract (UADT). A change in any of these three areas can change the quality of the voice.

The vibratory source creates a sound by chopping up air from the trachea by the intricate movement of the vocal cord mucosa. The vocal fold is a five-layered structure that allows the mucosa to move over Reinke's space and the lower elements that make up the vocal fold ligament. This movement is referred to as the mucosal wave and it forms a vibration that is then moulded by the UADT. The vocal folds may vibrate 80–1000 times/second; therefore, if visualized with white light, the mucosal wave cannot be visualized. Stroboscopic examination allows for the production of a montage of different phases in the cycle of the mucosal wave to be collected and visualized on screen. This chapter deals specifically with the history, examination and subsequent management of patients with abnormalities of the larynx.

HISTORY

When taking a history it is essential to listen carefully to the voice itself, as often a diagnosis can be made by listening to the quality of the voice and the story that comes with it.

It is essential to find out what the patient uses their voice for – both their occupation and their hobbies. Certain professions put more strain on their voices (e.g., teachers and actors) and are prone to pathology as a result.

The duration and progression of the hoarseness are important to ask about as longstanding voice changes are unlikely to be sinister, but a progressive change in the voice over a few months, especially associated with other UADT symptoms such as dysphagia, odynophagia, a neck mass or otalgia, indicates a potential malignant pathology.

Preceding symptoms, such as an upper respiratory tract infection (URTI), can affect the likelihood of pathology forming, especially in a situation where the voice is strained as a result of the URTI.

A thorough medical and drug history should be taken to assess conditions that may affect the ballast (respiratory drive) to produce voice. Also, certain medications may affect voice as they may precipitate coughing (ACEI's) or may dry the UADT (e.g., anticholinergic side-effects).

EXAMINATION

Initially, a general ENT examination is helpful, specifically looking at the oral cavity, oropharynx and nasal cavity, because these are the articulators and resonators and therefore affect voice.

Laryngeal examination then follows. The voice clinic often uses rigid laryngoscopy or flexible nasolaryngoscopy with a stack system. A stroboscopic light source allows the mucosal wave to be captured and processed by the human retina, enabling visualization of the differences between mucosal waves and also pathologies. Without a strobe the vibrations of the mucosal wave are too fast for the human retina to register. The strobe splits the wave up and puts together a cycle of its different aspects in a slower fashion for the retina to distinguish.

PATHOLOGY

Voice changes at the laryngeal level occur because of the following changes:

1 Mass effect on the vocal fold.
2 Incomplete closure of the vocal folds.

3 Poor vibration or mucosal wave as a result of pathology.

Common voice conditions and their treatment options are described below.

REINKE'S OEDEMA

In this situation the patient has had a long-standing deepening of the voice. They are often smokers, but acid reflux may also play a part. Pathologically, oedema occurs within Reinke's space in the vocal fold, increasing the mass of the vocal fold and therefore deepening the voice.

The correct treatment is smoking cessation and the use of anti-reflux therapy in the form of a proton pump inhibitor. If the patient ceases smoking but the voice does not return to normal and the findings are still the same on laryngoscopy, then a superior cordotomy on the non-vibratory surface of the vocal cord can be undertaken and some of the oedema reduced.

VOCAL FOLD NODULES ('SINGER'S' NODULES)

These are often associated with actors or singers, however, professional singers often have an excellent understanding of their voice and do not often present with nodules. Often the strain of pushing one's voice in inappropriate scenarios (i.e., acting or singing) can strain the voice and lead to trauma and the formation of nodules. Others (e.g., teachers and instructors in a noisy environment such as a swimming pool) may also suffer.

BILATERAL NODULES

The larynx often shows bilateral nodules at the junction of the anterior third and posterior two-thirds. This does not allow for good closure of the vocal folds and results in a change in voice.

For the vast majority of these we use speech and language therapy to educate the patient on use of the voice and to help them use their voice appropriately. Rarely do they require surgical intervention.

VOCAL FOLD PALSY

Patients present with a recent-onset, 'breathy' voice which becomes tired with use. The two vocal folds do not meet and therefore a lot of air escapes and a 'breathy' voice is created.

Sinister aetiology should be excluded as the nerve supply to the larynx is from the vagus via the recurrent laryngeal nerve. Imaging, including the skull base through to the upper chest, should be undertaken for a left cord palsy as the recurrent laryngeal nerve descends to the aortic arch on this side, and from skull base into the root of the neck for a right cord palsy (CT scan +/– MRI skull base).

Initially for an idiopathic vocal fold palsy speech and language therapy should be undertaken to see if the patient can compensate for the immobility and make the other cord come across further to make more contact and improve the voice. If this fails or for malignant aetiology (e.g., terminal lung cancer damaging the recurrent laryngeal nerve), speedier intervention is necessary. This requires an injection thyroplasty to medialize the immobile vocal cord, either as an outpatient or under general anaesthetic. An alternative is to medialize the vocal cord externally using a piece of silastic or Goretex through a window in the thyroid cartilage. (Pictures are required for injection thyroplasty under LA/GA and open thyroplasty.)

LARYNGEAL CANCER

These patients usually present with a long history of smoking and/or high alcohol intake. They have a progressively worsening voice over 6–12 weeks and may have associated otalgia, odynophagia, dysphagia and even associated neck lymphadenopathy.

Nasoendoscopy usually demonstrates an irregularity of the vocal fold but the patient requires a laryngoscopy and biopsy of this suspicious area. In smokers a premalignant diagnosis of dysplasia may be made on histology. This is just as important as the patient needs to be aware of this and stop smoking to reduce the chance of progressing to an invasive malignancy.

Laryngeal cancer can be treated in a variety of ways. Small laryngeal cancers can be treated with narrow field radiotherapy or be resected using a laser at the time of laryngoscopy. Larger tumours can be treated with radiotherapy or chemo-radiotherapy covering a larger field for associated lymph nodes. The largest laryngeal cancers – those that have invaded the thyroid cartilage – are often treated with a laryngectomy. This involves removal of the larynx and the creation of a permanent end stoma. The management of the patient should be discussed in the context of a multidisciplinary head and neck team meeting.

LARYNGEAL PAPILLOMATOSIS

Human papilloma virus (HPV) can cause viral warts. In the larynx this can be extremely troublesome. If a viral wart impinges the glottis, the airway may be compromised, but more often hoarseness is produced due to incomplete closure of the glottis and/or poor mucosal wave formation.

There are many treatments. Surgical interventions are often reserved for significant airway obstruction or for significant change in voice due to mass effect. The problem is that each surgical procedure is associated with some laryngeal scarring and although some patients will require multiple procedures it is wise to minimize the trauma to the larynx unless there is good reason to operate on it.

HAEMORRHAGIC POLYP

This pathology is not infrequently seen following an upper respiratory tract infection, where the voice has been used and then a small telangectatic vessel bleeds. This slight irregularity on the vocal cord leads to a change in voice. This sometimes heals, but occasionally persists and matures. If persistent, it may require surgical excision with a micro-laryngoscopy with or without laser resection.

VOCAL CORD GRANULOMA

Patients typically have undergone recent surgery requiring endotracheal intubation or have been on the Intensive Care Unit with an endotracheal tube *in situ* for a few days. The pathology forms typically on the posterior medial aspect of the vocal cord over the vocal process of the arytenoid cartilage. The granuloma forms due to healing exposed cartilage as a result of trauma from an endotracheal tube. Also of importance in the pathology may be gastropharyngeal reflux of acid.

Treatment often involves aggressive anti-reflux treatment over a six-week period, but if symptoms and signs persist, surgical resection may be undertaken with a micro-laryngoscopic technique.

VOCAL CORD CYSTS

This pathology presents clinically with a change in voice but it can be very variable in its severity and frequency. It may relate to the actual type of vocal cord cyst as some are superficial mucosal cysts and some are deeper intracordal cysts. These can be very difficult to treat and should be managed in a dedicated voice clinic, with full speech and language therapy support. However, if surgery is to be entertained, it should be carefully undertaken raising a microflap, dissecting the cyst out and causing minimal mucosal trauma. This should not be underestimated as it can prove to be a significant surgical challenge.

MICRO-LARYNGOSCOPY

This is an examination under general anaesthetia and is often undertaken for diagnostic or therapeutic procedures on the larynx. The use of the microscope offers magnification, depth of field, bimanual handling of instrumentation and the use of other attachments such as a CO_2 laser.

Before commencing a laryngoscopy the patient should be placed in 'the sniffing the morning air' position, which is flexion of the neck and extension of the atlanto-occipital joint. A decision on how to maintain the airway should be made with the anaesthetist (i.e., with a micro-laryngoscopy tube, supraglottic/subglottic or transtracheal jet ventilation).

The endoscope, light source, suction, lubrication and dental guard should all be checked prior to starting with the laryngoscopy. The laryngoscope is inserted carefully to get a view of the larynx and then suspended with a Lewis suspension arm. At this point the microscope or a Hopkins rod may be used for more careful examination of the larynx in preparation for the biopsy or surgical undertaking.

30 AIRWAY MANAGEMENT

Airway management is one of the most critical emergency situations in ENT practice. A sound understanding of the anatomy, physiology and management of a patient with airway problems is essential. In light of the order of resuscitation priorities – Airway, Breathing, Circulation (ABC) – the importance of airway management cannot be underestimated.

An additional point to consider is that as the airflow increases through a narrowed segment, pressure is decreased. This is known as the Bernoulli phenomenon. This draws the mucosa into an already narrowed airway inducing local oedema of the mucosa, which further narrows the airway with resulting compromise.

A further point to note is the difference between an adult's airway and a child's. In the child, the airway is both absolutely and relatively smaller than in the adult. The larynx is higher and external landmarks are less easily identifiable. The trachea lies nearer the skin in children, diving into the chest at a steeper angle than in the adult. Important contents of the thorax (e.g., the domes of the lungs and the great vessels) lie higher in the child. In addition, since the neonate is an obligatory nasal breather, nasal obstruction resulting from bilateral choanal atresia may be fatal.

MANAGEMENT OF THE COMPROMISED AIRWAY

Presentation and management of the compromised airway varies according to the site of presentation and aetiology (Table 30.1). These affect both the severity and speed of onset of symptoms and the categorization of management into urgent or non-urgent. However, the approach taken to manage airway obstruction is similar for all.

It is essential in the management of the patient with a compromised airway that a team approach is used. The most senior members of the anaesthetic and ENT teams should be informed and involved in the management at an early stage. More than one option or plan should be discussed before significant intervention is undertaken.

A rapid assessment of the patient is made to assess whether they are in danger of imminent upper airway obstruction. This is determined by the worsening of stridor or stertor, although stridor that becomes quiet may indicate imminent complete airway obstruction.

Stertor is rough noisy breathing, similar to snoring, caused by vibration of partially obstructing soft tissue in the pharynx.

Stridor is a harsh, high-pitched, almost musical sound, caused by vibration of partially obstructing soft tissue in the larynx or upper trachea.

Inspiratory stridor is during inspiration only, often a crowing sound, and is due to obstruction at the glottis, supraglottis or subglottis level.

Expiratory stridor is during expiration only, usually at a slightly lower pitch than inspiratory stridor, and is due to obstruction of the subglottis or extrathoracic trachea.

Biphasic stridor involves both inspiration and expiration, and, while representing laryngeal obstruction, is a hallmark of severe obstruction.

Wheeze is a high-pitched husky or whistling sound, caused by narrowing of soft tissue in the intrathoracic airways.

In addition, patients will have a high respiratory rate, poor chest expansion, low oxygen levels of saturations, tachycardia and may be tiring with rising carbon dioxide. The most common is obstruction in the larynx. While it may be possible in an adult to examine the larynx using a flexible nasoendoscope in order to assess the degree of obstruction, this must not be attempted in a child. When presented with a child with imminent airway compromise, such as suspected epiglottitis, never examine the child, take bloods or request an x-ray. The priority is to secure the airway, ideally in theatre. Any intervention may precipitate complete airway obstruction, which must be avoided. It is very rare that a patient presents in complete airway obstruction. In this case, it is likely that an anaesthetist will already be with the patient. If they are unable to intubate the patient, then an immediate tracheostomy must be performed in order to secure the airway. This is described in Chapter 28.

Immediate management includes calling for senior help, and giving oxygen and adrenaline nebulizers. Heliox can also buy valuable time. It is composed of 21% oxygen and 79% helium and has a lower density than air, which improves flow in the airways resulting in better oxygen delivery. The administration of steroids gives benefit a few hours later by reducing mucosal oedema. If in the emergency room, the patient should be monitored in the resuscitation area. If the patient is stable, they are managed in a high dependency or critical care unit. Where a patient is not severely compromised, a more thorough evaluation may be made, including appropriate imaging and a plan made depending on the aetiology.

If the patient is in complete airway obstruction or, despite the above measures, continues to deteriorate, then a decision must be taken to secure the airway with a cuffed endotracheal tube. Ideally, this should be performed in the operating theatre where all the anaesthetic equipment for managing difficult airways is available as well as the surgical instruments for tracheostomy and rigid bronchoscopes.

A plan is made jointly by the senior ENT surgeon and anaesthetist to determine how they will secure the airway. This depends on the suspected level of obstruction. Orotracheal or nasotracheal intubation may be attempted by the anaesthetist if it is thought that there is sufficient space to pass a tube through the obstruction safely. The surgeon and scrub nurse must be scrubbed with tracheostomy and bronchoscopes open and set up in order to intervene if needed. Other temporary airway adjuncts that should be considered to gain access to the subglottis include a transtracheal cannula or cricothyroidotomy with jet ventilation. If intubation fails or is thought not to be possible, then the decision is taken either to perform a tracheostomy or gain initial access to the airway by bronchoscopy with a rigid ventilating bronchoscope.

KEY POINTS:

1 A is for airway and the presentation of an acutely problematic airway is a medical and surgical emergency.
2 Act sooner rather than later, especially if you suspect a progressive problem.
3 Consider medical management that may be of use to hold the situation without causing the patient distress (adrenaline nebulizers, steroids, heliox).
4 Involve senior members of the ENT, anaesthetic and if appropriate nursing/paediatric teams as soon as possible.
5 Think before you act as you may precipitate a worsening of the problem.

Table 30.1 is a summary of the most common aetiologies that can result in airway obstruction along with the level of obstruction.

Table 30.1. Aetiology of airway obstruction.

Level of obstruction	Aetiology	
	Pathological	**Anatomical**
Nasopharynx	Tumour Infection Foreign body	Choanal atresia (unilateral or bilateral) Crouzon's disease Apert's syndrome
Oropharynx/ Hypopharynx	Infection (tonsillitis, Ludwig's angina) Bleeding (post-tonsillectomy) Tumour Burns Trauma Anaphylaxis	Short lower jaw (especially micrognathia) Large tongue
Supraglottis	Infection (epiglotitis, supraglottitis) Bleeding Tumour (squamous cell carcinoma, respiratory papillomatosis) Cyst of vallecular or epiglottis Anaphylaxis Foreign body	Laryngomalacia
Glottis	Infection (croup) Tumour (squamous cell carcinoma, respiratory papillomatosis) Vocal cord palsy Polyp Oedema (postoperative anaphylaxis) Foreign body	Laryngeal cleft Laryngeal web
Subglottis	Infection (croup) Tumour (squamous cell carcinoma, respiratory papillomatosis) Stricture (post-intubation, post-tracheostomy) Extrinsic compression (thyroid, lymph nodes, tumour) Foreign body	Congenital subglottic stenosis Subglottic haemangioma
Tracheal	Infection (tracheitis) Tumour (squamous cell carcinoma, respiratory papillomatosis Stricture (post-tracheostomy) Foreign body Bleeding (post-tracheostomy) Burns	Tracheosophageal fistula

31 RADIOLOGY

LATERAL SOFT TISSUE FILM

This is a plain x-ray performed in the acute setting for investigation of an ingested foreign body in an adult or child. A normal lateral soft tissue film is illustrated in Figure 31.1.

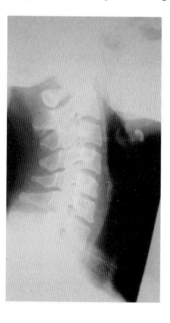

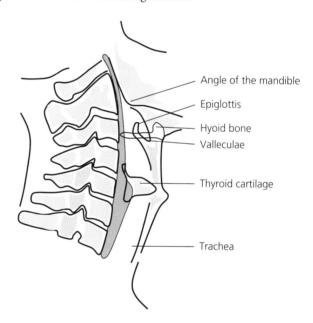

Figure 31.1. Landmarks visible on a lateral soft tissue film of the neck. The soft tissue space anterior to the vertebral column should always be inspected.

Always check for prevertebral soft tissue swelling.

The maximum normal width anterior to the upper cervical vertebral bodies (C1–C4) should measure up to 7 mm. The maximal normal width increases to 22 mm in the lower cervical vertebrae (C5–C7). This is more easily estimated by remembering that up to a third of the vertebral body is allowed between C1–C4 and a whole vertebral body's width is allowed anterior to C5–C7.

There is a wide variety in the radio density of swallowed foreign bodies. Whilst some ingested foreign bodies are radio-opaque and clearly visible on a lateral soft tissue film, many are not. Helpful secondary radiological signs that suggest the presence of an impacted foreign body include widening of the prevertebral soft tissue space (as a result of surgical emphysema due to perforation or retropharyngeal abscess formation), tenting of the cervical oesophagus producing a gas shadow in the upper cervical oesophagus or straightening of the normal cervical lordosis.

Common sites for impingement of chicken or fish bones include the palatine tonsils, tongue base, valleculae and pyriform fossae. The oesophagus is narrowed just below the level of the cricopharyngeus and at the level of the aortic arch. It is here that foreign bodies are commonly located.

A normal soft tissue lateral film cannot exclude a radiolucent foreign body and a low threshold should be maintained for endoscopy. Similarly, normal variants with calcification within the cricoid or arytenoids can be mistaken for bones due to their curvilinear calcification.

A chest x-ray may be an alternative test if the suspected level of the obstruction is in the thoracic oesophagus or airways.

Common sites of oesophageal foreign body impaction are:

- At the level of the cricopharyngeus.
- Where the arch of the aorta indents the oesophagus.
- Where the right main bronchus indents the oesophagus.
- At the cardiac sphincter.

CONTRAST SWALLOW

A contrast swallow may be indicated for the following:

- Globus sensation.
- Suspected pharyngeal pouch.
- Suspected foreign body.
- Suspected oesophageal lesion.

The barium or contrast swallow is a fluoroscopic technique using low-dose pulsed x-rays to examine the pharynx and oesophagus. It can be used to demonstrate strictures, tumours, pharyngeal pouches, tracheo-oesophageal fistulae, oesophageal dysmotility and gastro-oesophageal reflux. A non-ionic contrast medium such as Omnipaque is used in cases where there is a clinical suspicion of aspiration as barium can remain in the chest indefinitely and alternatives such as gastrograffin can cause a chemical pneumonitis.

ULTRASOUND NECK

Ultrasound is a safe, easily accessible test. Superficial structures such as the thyroid, parotid and submandibular glands are easily evaluated and beautifully depicted. Morphology of lymph nodes and the presence of any suspicious features, as well as diagnostic fine needle aspiration (FNA), can be performed. The presence of collections and whether they would be amenable to drainage can be determined. In children it can be used to assess lesions such as thyroglossal cysts or fibromatosis colli (sternomastoid tumour). The presence or absence and velocity of coloured blood flow in congenital lesions such as venolymphatic malformations and haemangiomas can be assessed as an adjunct to further cross-sectional imaging, such as MRI.

CT AXIAL VIEWS OF THE NECK

CT of the neck is usually performed in the acute setting for assessing adenopathy or a collection. MRI is better at delineating soft tissue planes and has no ionizing burden, but availability in the acute setting is limited and scanning times can be lengthy for the improved spatial resolution required for the small structures in the neck.

CT OF THE TEMPORAL BONE

CT of the temporal bone is used as a preoperative planning tool in cases of cholesteatoma where disease spread resulting in bony erosion is particularly significant (Figure 31.2). The bony ossicular chain and inner ear can be assessed as well as the aeration of the surrounding mastoid air cells. It is also useful in cases where hyperostosis is seen as a complication of meningitis.

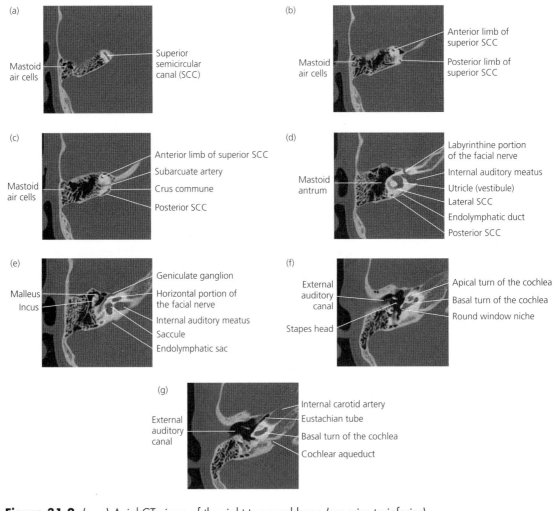

Figure 31.2. (a–g) Axial CT views of the right temporal bone (superior to inferior).

A CT scan is reviewed in order specifically to assess:

- Extent of disease.
- Pneumatization of the temporal bone.
- Position of the sigmoid sinus.
- Facial nerve dehiscence.
- Position and dehiscence of the tegmen/middle fossa plate.
- Ossicular chain continuity.
- A breach of the inner ear.

CT OF THE SINUSES

CT of the sinuses has now replaced plain film radiography and is indicated in patients who do not respond to medical treatment of sinusitis. It can demonstrate severity and distribution of disease, patency of the osteo-meatal complexes and any anatomical variants such as concha bullosa (an accessory air cell within the middle turbinate), Haller and Onodi cells and to aid surgery. Both coronal sections and axial sections are required.

A CT scan is reviewed in order specifically to assess:

1 Extent of disease.
2 Position of the septum – a deviated septum may require correction in order to access the parana-sal sinuses (Figure 31.3).
3 Position of lamina papyracea and uncinate process.
4 Attachment of the middle turbinate.
5 Presence of a concha bullosae.
6 Length of the lateral lemniscus (Keros classification; Table 31.1).
7 Position of the optic nerves (axial views).

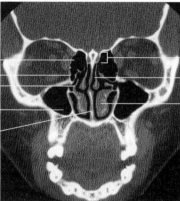

Anterior ethmoidal air cell
Lamina papyracea
Uncinate process
Maxillary sinus
Septum
Lateral lemniscus
Middle turbinate
Inferior turbinate

Figure 31.3. Coronal section of the paranasal sinuses.

Table 31.1. The Keros classification refers to the vertical height of the lateral lemniscus. Types 2 and 3 are at greater risk of CSF leak during functional endoscopic sinus surgery.

	Vertical height of the lateral lemniscus
Type 1	1–3 mm
Type 2	4–7 mm
Type 3	8–16 mm

MAGNETIC RESONANCE IMAGING

Indications

- Assessment of the tongue base.
- Assessment of parotid lesions.
- Intracranial pathology (e.g., CPA lesions).

MRI is increasingly used in the head and neck due to its capacity to image the soft tissues. This modal-ity remains the investigation of choice in the assess-ment of tongue base or parotid lesions. In the case of the latter, the retromandibular vein allows one to distinguish between the larger superficial and smaller deep lobe tumours. The extent of tongue carcinoma is best defined radiologically, with particular regard to whether the midline has been crossed, whether there is involvement of the mandible and any spread posteriorly to the epiglottis.

▌ MRI IAMs

Normal anatomy, including the VIIth and VIIIth nerve roots and the vestibular aqueduct, are exquisitely demonstrated.

Most ENT surgeons will request this investigation for cases of asymmetric sensorineural hearing loss (>15 dB HL difference in two adjacent frequencies), sudden sensorineural hearing loss and unexplained vertigo or dizziness. It may also be used to assess patients with delayed or absent recovery of a facial nerve paralysis.

This investigation is contraindicated in patients with metal foreign bodies and implants (e.g., pacemakers, cochlear implants, etc.).

Both high-resolution CT and MRI are important in the investigation of congenital deafness as well as the surgical planning of any treatment. There is a wide range of anatomical abnormalities, some linked to syndromes, including the Mondini spectrum and widening of the vestibular aqueduct.

32 MANAGEMENT OF NECK LUMPS

The management of masses in the head and neck region may seem daunting because of the wide variety of pathology and the consequences of missing an important diagnosis. This exceptionally common clinical finding can be seen across the age groups and important factors must be elicited in order to obtain the correct diagnosis.

An understanding of the anatomy of the neck and the associated pathologies relevant to the various positions in the neck is helpful. Delineation of whether a lump is in the midline (often suggestive of a thyroid or thyroglossal cyst pathology) or laterally, either in the anterior or posterior triangle of the neck, can assist in the diagnosis.

HISTORY

A careful history should be elicited from the patient. Age of onset of the neck lump should be documented as congenital pathology presents in the early years and more often malignant pathologies present later in life. Upper aero-digestive tract symptoms, such as dysphonia, dysphagia, odynophagia, otalgia and breathing disorders, can be helpful in localizing pathology. Personal habits such as smoking and high alcohol intake can highlight a risk for malignant potential.

EXAMINATION

A thorough examination of the head and neck should be undertaken. The oral cavity should be illuminated with a headlight and examined with two tongue depressors. If appropriate, the tongue base should be palpated as pathology may be deep and not obvious to the eye (this does, however, induce a significant gag reflex). A flexible fibre-optic nasolaryngoscope is usually required to assess the postnasal space, larynx and hypopharynx. Any masses in the neck should be identified in a careful and methodical examination of the neck.

SPECIAL INVESTIGATIONS

The use of special investigations can be divided into those pertinent to preparing a patient for a general anaesthetic and those relevant to the pathology of the head and neck.

When investigating a lump in the neck the principal investigation of choice, almost always, is fine needle aspirate cytology (FNAC). This is a process by which cells are sampled by means of multiple passes of a needle through the mass while simultaneously aspirating with a syringe. The cells in the barrel of the needle are then sprayed onto a cytology slide and either air-dried or fixed chemically, depending on the preference of the cytology department. This test is often undertaken by the cytology department itself. This is a crucial investigation and there are only a few instances where an FNAC of a neck lump is not appropriate.

Imaging of masses in the neck is commonplace. The choice of imaging is dependent on the patient and the institution where it is to be performed. Ultrasonography is an excellent, non-invasive tool to delineate structures but is difficult to interpret by the surgeon. Computerized tomography (CT) is superb at looking at most of the head and neck, is easy to obtain and quick to undertake, but can be prone to dental artefact in and around the oral cavity. Magnetic resonance imaging (MRI) is an excellent tool to look at soft tissues, especially of the tongue, postnasal space and oral cavity. It does often carry a longer waiting time to be performed, is more claustrophobic to have undertaken and takes longer to be scanned.

Investigations pertinent to general anaesthesia should be discussed at a local preadmission level and each department should have an appropriate protocol for preparing a patient for general anaesthesia.

TREATMENT

The treatment of any neck mass is dependent on the diagnosis. Reactive lymphadenopathy secondary to tonsillitis requires treatment of the tonsillitis with antibiotics. Congenital pathologies may be observed if asymptomatic but, if causing problems, often warrant surgical excision. The primary malignant disease of the upper aero-digestive tract may be treated with surgery, radiotherapy, chemo-radiotherapy or a combination of these. All treatment plans will be decided in the context of a multidisciplinary team meeting.

LYMPHADENOPATHY

Lymphadenopathy can be benign or malignant. The benign causes of lymphadenopathy are multiple and too large a group to be discussed in this chapter. However, a lymph node in the neck should be approached as though it is malignant until it is shown that it is not. Our index of suspicion is changed by different aspects of the history, clinical examination and special investigations performed. Metastatic lymphadenopathy typically follows a predictable path dependent on the primary site of the tumour (Figure 32.1). This should be borne in mind when searching for the primary tumour. Lymphoma is a diagnosis that should be considered but is difficult to diagnose on FNAC. Often a lymph node biopsy is required for formal exclusion or typing of the lymphoma.

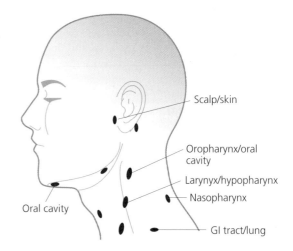

Figure 32.1. Metastatic spread from primary sites in head and neck cancer.

THYROGLOSSAL DUCT CYST

This congenital anomaly occurs due to residual portions of the tract that forms during the descent of the thyroid gland during embryological development. The cysts can form at any point along the descent of the thyroid and are often found in a paramedian position, between the trachea and the base of tongue.

These should be investigated with an ultrasound scan to look at the mass, but also to check for a normal thyroid gland, as surgical excision is often contemplated and one must be certain there is other thyroid tissue left behind after its removal.

Surgery is in the form of a Sistrunk's procedure or midline neck dissection clearing the tissue from the midline of the neck and the cyst whilst taking out the mid-portion of the hyoid bone. Removal of the mid-portion of the hyoid bone is undertaken due to the intimacy of the embryological descent with the hyoid and its removal significantly decreases the recurrence rate of these cysts.

BRANCHIAL CYST

Branchial cysts are another congenital pathology that typically present in the first two decades of life. They may present as an asymptomatic mass but can be seen to enlarge, especially in association with upper respiratory tract infections. The position of these is quite characteristic, being hidden under the junction of the upper third and lower two-thirds of the sternocleidomastoid muscle.

FNAC often demonstrates a straw-coloured liquid. Imaging should be undertaken in the form of a CT or MRI scan of the neck to give relationships to the great vessels and also to characterize the mass further.

Surgical excision should not be undertaken lightly and should be considered almost like a selective neck dissection, such that the accessory, hypoglossal and vagus nerves are identified and preserved together with the internal jugular vein and the carotid artery.

THYROID MASSES

Thyroid masses are commonplace and warrant a whole chapter. However, certain aspects of the history should be elicited, namely aspects of the lump and growth rate, pain, dysphagia, hoarseness and stridor, together with aspects of risk factors, such a family history or exposure to ionizing radiation.

Many people argue about investigation of the thyroid mass. This depends on the institution's expertise; however, most people with a mass in the thyroid will have at least an ultrasound and FNAC to guide the surgeon in their management plan.

Treatment is dependent on the appearances of the FNAC and ultrasound, together with the patient's feeling about the lump, as cosmesis is an indication for removal of a goitre.

SALIVARY GLAND TUMOURS

This is an extensive subject, but it is useful to have an understanding of it.

Eighty per cent of salivary gland tumours arise in the parotid, 10% in the submandibular gland and

10% in the sublingual or minor salivary glands. Of the parotid tumours 80% are benign and of these 80% are pleomorphic adenomas.

Hallmark symptoms and signs of malignant pathology include rapid growth of mass, pain and nerve weakness (e.g., facial nerve weakness in parotid malignancies).

FNAC is very useful and can be very helpful in the decision-making process for these tumours.

33 VERTIGO AND DIZZINESS

Vertigo and dizziness affect approximately a third of the general population before the age of 65 years, and approximately two-thirds of women and one third of men at 80 years (1). Annually, 5/1000 patients present to their general practitioner complaining of vertigo, and another 10/1000 with symptoms of dizziness or giddiness (2). A balance disorder in the elderly may result in a fall, and the subsequent injuries sustained leading to death in this age group (3, 4, 5).

BALANCE OVERVIEW

Normal human balance relies on vision, proprioception and the peripheral vestibular organs (Figure 33.1). This sensory information is relayed centrally, and integrated and interpreted within the

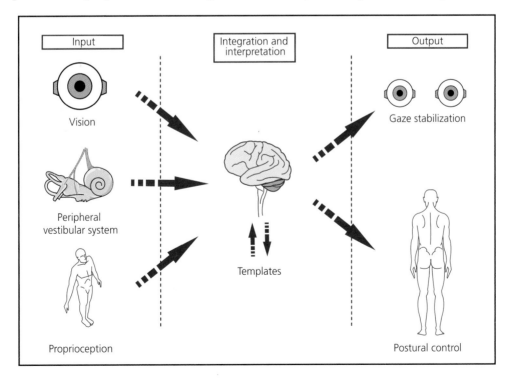

Figure 33.1. Overview of the balance system.

brain in order to maintain posture and stabilize vision. Interpretation involves cross-referencing this sensory information with previously generated templates. A mismatch results in symptoms of dizziness, unsteadiness or vertigo.

HISTORY

Taking a thorough history is the key to establishing a diagnosis. It is essential to allow a patient to speak freely at the start of the consultation. Although some of this information may be of little diagnostic value, it does allow some insight into their principal concerns and also establishes rapport with the patient. It is often the case that this will be the first time that 'anyone has listened'.

A detailed history of the first episode is essential. When, where and what possible precipitants were associated with this event should be sought. The duration and form of dizziness/vertigo should also be established. Associated symptoms should be documented (e.g., nausea, vomiting, hearing loss, tinnitus, loss of consciousness, photophobia, headache).

Subsequent episodes, their duration, frequency and precipitants, will confirm a working diagnosis. The most recent episode is also worth exploring as symptoms may evolve as central changes partially compensate for the peripheral or central pathology. It is always worth considering more than a single pathology to be responsible for a patient's symptoms (e.g., benign paroxysmal positional vertigo (BPPV) and a peripheral vestibular deficit).

A past medical and surgical history must always be taken. This must include details regarding the patient's vision and mobility, and a family or personal history of migraine must always be explored. In females, a delicate and difficult subject is that of spontaneous miscarriage, but may suggest an autoimmune or embolic aetiology. A note should be made of previous or current anxiety or depression (6).

EXAMINATION

A full neuro-otological examination is required in every patient presenting with vertigo. Although a working diagnosis may have been made it is essential both to confirm and exclude possible concurrent pathology. This includes cranial nerve examination, eye movement in all four planes for nystagmus, smooth pursuit, saccades, latent squint, and assessment for cerebellar signs. Romberg's test (on both floor and foam) and Fukuda step testing should also be performed. Whilst the latter is generally regarded to localize a peripheral vestibular deficit (rotation occurs towards the weaker side), the Halmagyi head thrust test is a far more sensitive and specific

clinical investigation (7). Dix-Hallpike testing is also required in every case to demonstrate any form of nystagmus, but in particular geotropic torsional nystagmus consistent with posterior semicircular canal BPPV (8). Vertical or horizontal nystagmus, or nystagmus that does not fatigue, is unusual and patients require MRI scanning to exclude central pathology. It is essential to document the latency and duration of any nystagmus seen and whether the nystagmus settled completely.

A thorough assessment also includes lying and standing blood pressure recording and functional gait assessment.

SPECIAL INVESTIGATIONS

All patients must undergo a pure tone audiogram and tympanometry. A sensorineural asymmetry may suggest a cerebellopontine angle tumour, which must therefore be excluded. A full audio-vestibular battery is required in the majority of subjects referred to a balance service (exceptions may include BPPV that settles completely following particle repositioning manoeuvres). Not only do these investigations support a working diagnosis, but in approximately 5–10% of cases reveal unexpected unilateral or bilateral peripheral vestibular hypofunction.

As it is not possible to directly access the peripheral vestibular organs, an indirect assessment based on the vestibulo-ocular reflex is generally used (Figure 33.2).

Bithermal caloric testing remains a simple and valuable method of comparing lateral semicircular

function. Eye movements may be recorded with electrodes attached to the face, electronystagmography (ENG), or by videoing pupil movement, videonystagmography (VNG). Saccades, smooth pursuit and optikokinetic movement may also be assessed with this recording method. Additional tests include rotational chair and vestibular evoked myogenic potentials (VEMPs).

Patients with a history and assessment in keeping with central pathology should also undergo an MRI scan to exclude a space-occupying lesion or demyelination. Patients with chronic ear disease or suspected superior semicircular canal dehiscence require a fine-cut computed tomography scan of the temporal bones.

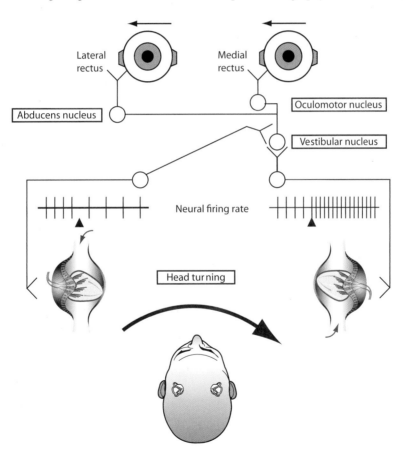

Figure 33.2. The vestibulo-ocular reflex. As a result of head rotation, endolymph flow within the semicircular canals causes movement of the cupulae within the ampullae of the lateral semicircular canals and relative shearing of the underlying stereocilia. Neural impulses increase on the right and decrease on the left. Neural connections to the IIIrd and VIth cranial nuclei result in contraction of the left lateral rectus and right medial rectus to stabilize gaze.

COMMON VESTIBULAR PATHOLOGY

Listed below are common vestibular conditions amenable to treatment (Table 33.1). Management pathways are also illustrated in Figure 33.3.

Benign paroxysmal positional vertigo (BPPV)

This is the commonest cause of vertigo in all age groups. Patients classically describe rotatory vertigo when rising or turning over in bed. Although the vertigo lasts for seconds, they feel unsteady for a great deal longer, but are then able to go about their normal daily activities. There is no associated hearing loss or tinnitus. Spells last for days to weeks and usually settle spontaneously. Patients invariably, though not universally, describe a previous head injury or an episode of 'labyrinthitis'.

Symptoms arise due to debris derived from the otoconial membrane of the utricle. Head rotation results in this debris striking the delicate cupula of the posterior semicircular canal, profoundly stimulating the associated hair cells and causing vertigo (Figure 33.2). The mismatch that occurs may also result in nausea, vomiting and anxiety.

In the most common form, posterior canal BPPV, on Dix-Hallpike testing, following a short latency, geotropic torsional nystagmus will gradually appear, increase in severity and subside completely. This will correlate well with the symptoms of vertigo experienced by the patient during the test. Having confirmed the diagnosis, an Epley manoeuvre should be performed. This is curative in approximately 90% of cases. A repeat manoeuvre may on occasion be required. Alternative particle repositioning manoeuvres for posterior semicircular canal BBPV include Brandt-Daroff (9) and Semont (10) manoeuvres. Gan's manoeuvre may be used if the anterior semicircular canal is involved (11).

Acute peripheral vestibular deficit (labyrinthitis/vestibular neuritis)

This relatively common cause of vertigo arises due to a sudden failure of one peripheral vestibular organ. This results in labyrinthine asymmetry, and the sensory mismatch that occurs causes severe persistent rotatory vertigo and profuse vomiting.

Patients frequently describe a recent flu-like illness. They classically wake with severe continuous rotatory vertigo that persists for 3–5 days. Initially, patients must lie still as any movement results in worsening symptoms. Thereafter, movements may be tolerated but compensation for normal activities may take weeks or months. Prochlorperazine, a peripheral vestibular sedative, is indicated in such situations but should be limited to seven days as long-term use may limit central compensation and hence functional recovery.

Clinical examination may reveal rotation on Fukuda step testing. More reliable is the head thrust test, where a catch-up saccade may be evident.

Patients who do not compensate, benefit from generic or customized physiotherapy. Those with visual vertigo (over-reliance on visual input) benefit from combining physiotherapy exercises and visually stimulating environments (12). Those who fail to improve must be reassessed and possible limitations to compensation excluded (Table 33.2).

Vertiginous migraine

Also known as migraine variant, this common cause of vertigo produces spells of vertigo or dysequilibrium that last for several days and in women are frequently associated with menstruation. Patients often describe phonophobia or photophobia and prefer to rest in a quiet,

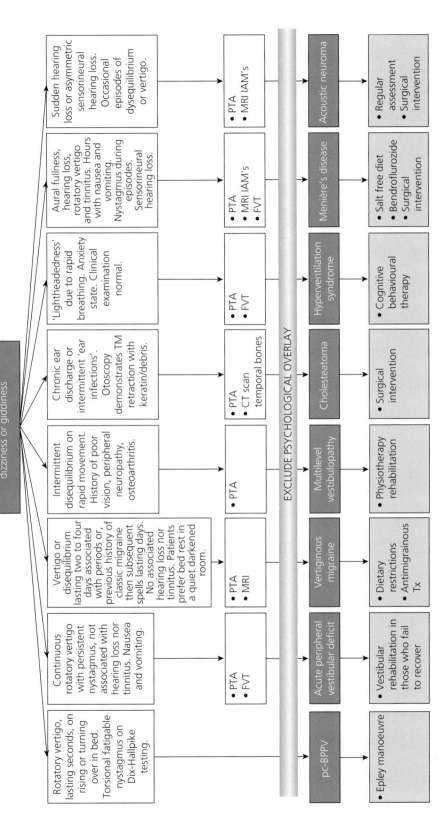

Figure 33.3. Management pathways for common vestibular pathology. (PTA–pure tone audiometry, FVT–formal vestibular testing).

Table 33.1. Common causes of dizziness (in order of frequency).

- Benign paroxysmal positional vertigo (BPPV)
- Labyrinthitis/vestibular neuritis
- Vertiginous migraine
- Multilevel vestibulopathy
- Cholesteatoma (CSOM)
- Hyperventilation syndrome
- Menière's disease
- Acoustic neuroma
- Multiple sclerosis
- Vertebro-basillar insufficiency
- Superior semicircular canal dehiscence

darkened room. There is no associated hearing loss nor tinnitus.

Although no abnormalities are likely to be found on clinical examination, ENG/VNG testing may support central changes. All patients should undergo MRI scanning in order to exclude central pathology.

Treatment consists of dietary changes (avoidance of chocolate, caffeine, red wine, cheese and processed meat). The majority of patients benefit from this approach alone, although some may also require

tricyclic antidepressants, calcium channel blockers or beta-blockers.

▌ Multilevel vestibulopathy

Dizziness and vertigo are common symptoms in elderly patients.

Unilateral decline in one sensory pathway may be compensated for centrally with little or no functional loss. A reduction in the quality and quantity of sensory information from multiple sensory pathways, in addition to central changes within the brain (e.g., ischaemic episodes) may result in multilevel vestibulopathy. Patients benefit from a combination of physiotherapy exercises (generic, customized or strength and balance exercises) and lifestyle changes (e.g., the use of a walking stick, visual acuity/cataract correction).

▌ Cholesteatoma (CSOM)

Squamous epithelium within the middle ear may expand to erode into the inner ear. While most patients present with intermittent or chronic ear discharge, with hearing loss, some also complain of intermittent vertigo and unsteadiness.

Table 33.2. Limitations of vestibular compensation.

Visual impairment	Cataracts Poor visual acuity Eye movement disorders Visual impairment
Peripheral vestibular system	Prolonged vestibular sedative use (e.g., prochlorperazine) Recurrent or progressive vestibular insults
Proprioception	Immobility
Psychological factors	Anxiety Depression Agoraphobia
Central pathology	Cerebrovascular disease Intracranial pathology
Rehabilitation	Delay in starting vestibular rehabilitation Poor motivation
Concurrent illness	

Hyperventilation syndrome

Hyperventilation, associated with anxiety, may result in light-headedness and dizziness. In some, anxiety may be the residual effect of a previous vestibular insult which the patient may have compensated for. Symptoms can be reproduced by asking a patient to breathe rapidly through pursed lips. Such patients benefit from a cognitive behavioural therapy review.

Menière's disease

Previously over-diagnosed, this rare cause for vertigo arises due to mixing of perilymph and endolymph within the inner ear. This results in an initial feeling of aural fullness followed by hearing loss, severe rotatory vertigo and tinnitus.

Attacks are unpredictable and severe. A pure tone audiogram will demonstrate a sensorineural hearing loss, initially in the low frequencies in the affected ear and then, as attacks continue, hearing loss across all frequencies. It is essential to exclude a central pathology (e.g., a cerebello-pontine angle tumour) and hence an MRI scan must be performed. Bithermal calorics will reveal a peripheral vestibular weakness. Attacks eventually subside, but at the expense of the hearing in the affected ear.

Treatment includes Buccastem for acute episodes, and bendrofluorazide or betahistine to reduce the frequency and severity of attacks.

For those not controlled medically, surgery may be indicated. Procedures include grommet insertion, gentamicin ablation, medical or surgical labyrinthectomy and vestibular nerve section.

Other relatively uncommon conditions that may present with vertigo or dizziness include multiple sclerosis, acoustic neuroma (Figure 33.4) and vertebro-basillar ischaemia. In each an MRI scan is required to establish a diagnosis.

Superior semicircular canal dehiscence is a rare condition whereby a defect in the bony covering of the superior semicircular canal results in a third window through which a pressure wave may be

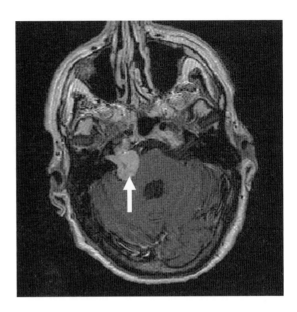

Figure 33.4. Right acoustic neuroma.

transmitted from and to the intracranial cavity. This not only results in momentary vertigo in response to loud sounds (Tullio's phenomenon), but also results in patients hearing their eyes moving.

KEY POINTS:

1 An understanding of the sensory pathways and their central interpretation provides a valuable guide to the diagnosis and management of patients who complain of vertigo and dizziness.
2 While a number of conditions exist that may result in vertiginous spells, treatment is either curative or enormously beneficial in the vast majority of patients.
3 The commonest cause of vertigo, BPPV, should be excluded in all cases by Dix-Hallpike testing.

REFERENCES
1 Shepard NT, Telian SA (1996a). Balance Disorder Patient. Basic Anatomy and Physiology Review. Singular Publishing Group, Inc.

2 The Royal College of General Practitioners and Office of Population Census and Surveys (1986). Morbidity Statistics from General Practice. HMSO, London.

3 Blake AJ, Morgan K, Bendall MJ *et al* (1988). Falls by elderly people at home: Prevalence and associated factors. Age and Ageing **17**: 365–72.

4 Campbell AJ, Reinken J, Allan BC, Martinez GS (1981). Falls in old age: A study of frequency and related clinical factors. Age and Ageing **10**: 264–70.

5 Stevens JA, Olson S (2000). Reducing falls and resulting hip fractures among older women. *MMWR Recomm Rep* **49**: 3–12.

6 McKenna L, Hallam RS, Hinchcliffe R (1991). The prevalence of psychological disturbance in neuro-otology outpatients. *Clinical Otolaryngology* **16**: 452–6.

7 Halmagyi GM, Curthoys IS (1988). A clinical sign of canal paresis. *Archives of Neurology* **45**: 737–9.

8 Dix, R, Hallpike C (1952). The pathology, symptomatology and diagnosis of certain common disorders of the vestibular system. *Annals of Otology, Rhinology and Laryngology* **6**: 987–1016.

9 Brandt T, Daroff R (1980). Physical therapy for benign paroxysmal positional vertigo. *Archives of Otolaryngology* **106**: 484–5.

10 Semont A, Freyss G, Vitte E (1988). Curing the BPPV with a liberatory maneuver. *Advances in Otorhinolaryngology* **42**: 290–3.

11 Gans R (2000). Overview of BPPV: Treatment methodologies. *Hearing Review* **7**: 50–4.

12 Pavlou M, Lingeswaran A., Davies RA, *et al* (2004). Simulator based rehabilitation in refractory dizziness. *J Neurol* **251**: 983–95.

INDEX